The Washington Manual™ Psychiatry Survival Guide

D0814064

The Washington Manual™ Psychiatry Survival Guide

Editor

Keith S. Garcia, M.D., Ph.D.
Instructor of Psychiatry
Washington University School of Medicine
St. Louis, Missouri

Series Editor

Tammy L. Lin, M.D.
Adjunct Assistant Professor of Medicine
Washington University School of Medicine
St. Louis, Missouri

Series Advisor

Daniel M. Goodenberger, M.D.
Professor of Medicine
Chief, Division of Medical Education
Washington University School of Medicine
Director, Internal Medicine Residency
   Program
Barnes-Jewish Hospital
St. Louis, Missouri

LIPPINCOTT WILLIAMS & WILKINS
A **Wolters Kluwer** Company
Philadelphia • Baltimore • New York • London
Buenos Aires • Hong Kong • Sydney • Tokyo

Acquisitions Editor: Danette Knopp
Developmental Editors: Scott Marinaro and Keith Donnellan
Supervising Editor: Allison Risko
Production Editor: Amanda Waltman Yanovitch, Silverchair Science + Communications
Manufacturing Manager: Colin Warnock
Cover Designer: QT Design
Compositor: Silverchair Science + Communications
Printer: Victor Graphics

© 2003 by Department of Medicine, Washington University School of Medicine

Printed in the USA

Library of Congress Cataloging-in-Publication Data
Garcia, Keith S.
  The Washington manual psychiatry survival guide / Keith S. Garcia.
    p. ; cm. -- (Washington manual survival guide series)
  Includes bibliographical references and index.
  ISBN 0-7817-4367-2
    1. Psychiatry--Handbooks, manuals, etc. 2. Mental illness--Diagnosis--Handbooks, manuals, etc. I. Title: Manual psychiatry survival guide. II. North, Carol S. III. Title. IV. Series.
  [DNLM: 1. Mental Disorders--diagnosis--Handbooks. 2. Internship and Residency--Handbooks. 3. Psychiatry--methods--Handbooks. WM 34 G261w 2003]
RC456.G37 2003
616.89--dc21
                                                                      2003050102

The Washington Manual™ is an intent-to-use mark belonging to Washington University in St. Louis to which international legal protection applies. The mark is used in this publication by LWW under license from Washington University.

Care has been taken to confirm the accuracy of the information presented and to describe generally accepted practices. However, the authors, editors, and publisher are not responsible for errors or omissions or for any consequences from application of the information in this book and make no warranty, expressed or implied, with respect to the currency, completeness, or accuracy of the contents of the publication. Application of this information in a particular situation remains the professional responsibility of the practitioner.

The authors, editors, and publisher have exerted every effort to ensure that drug selection and dosage set forth in this text are in accordance with current recommendations and practice at the time of publication. However, in view of ongoing research, changes in government regulations, and the constant flow of information relating to drug therapy and drug reactions, the reader is urged to check the package insert for each drug for any change in indications and dosage and for added warnings and precautions. This is particularly important when the recommended agent is a new or infrequently employed drug.

Some drugs and medical devices presented in this publication have Food and Drug Administration (FDA) clearance for limited use in restricted research settings. It is the responsibility of health care providers to ascertain the FDA status of each drug or device planned for use in their clinical practice.

10 9 8 7 6 5 4 3 2

Contents

Chairman's Note

Medical knowledge is increasing at an exponential rate, and physicians are being bombarded with new facts at a pace that many find overwhelming. The Washington Manual™ Survival Guides were developed in this context for interns, residents, medical students, and other practitioners in need of readily accessible practical clinical information. They therefore meet an important need in an era of information overload.

I would like to acknowledge the authors who have contributed to these books. In particular, Tammy L. Lin, M.D., Series Editor, provided energetic and inspired leadership, and Daniel M. Goodenberger, M.D., Series Advisor, Chief of the Division of Medical Education in the Department of Medicine at Washington University, is a continual source of sage advice. The efforts and outstanding skill of the lead authors are evident in the quality of the final product. I am confident that this series will meet its desired goal of providing practical knowledge that can be directly applied to improving patient care.

Kenneth S. Polonsky
Adolphus Busch Professor
Chairman, Department of Medicine
Washington University School of Medicine
St. Louis, Missouri

Series Preface

The Washington Manual™ Survival Guides, a multispecialty series, is designed to provide interns, residents, medical students, or anyone on the front lines of clinical care with quick, practical, and essential information in an accessible format. It lets you hit the ground running as you learn the basics of practicing clinical medicine, gain more responsibility, and become a valued team member. Although written individually, they all incorporate series features. Each book takes care to give you an insider's view of how to get things done efficiently and effectively, tips on how to "survive" training, and pearls you will want to pass on in the future. It is similar to receiving a great sign-out from your favorite resident. When faced with an unfamiliar situation, we envision getting timely information and guidance from the survival guide (like you would from your resident) to make appropriate decisions at 3:00 p.m. or 3:00 a.m.

One of the most unique and notable features of this new series is that it was truly a joint effort across subspecialties at Washington University. We were fortunate to have significant departmental support, particularly from Kenneth Polonsky, M.D., whose commitment made this series possible. Every survival guide has the credibility of being written by recent interns, residents, or chief residents in that specialty with input from faculty advisors. We were fortunate to have found outstanding head authors who were not only highly regarded clinicians and teachers, but who also provided significant leadership and collaborated well together. Their incredible enthusiasm and desire to pass on their hard-earned knowledge, experiences, and wisdom clearly shines through in the series.

Anyone who has been through training will tell you the hours are long, the work is hard, and your energy is limited. With either a print or electronic version of a survival guide by your side, we hope you will work more efficiently, make decisions with more confidence, stay out of trouble, and get that ever-elusive good night's rest.

Tammy L. Lin, M.D., Series Editor
Daniel M. Goodenberger, M.D., Series Advisor

Preface

This is the first edition of *The Washington Manual™ Psychiatry Survival Guide,* a pocket book intended to provide a quick reference for the hospital practice of psychiatric medicine in the inpatient psychiatric, consultation, and emergency settings. Each section provides abstracted information on the most frequently encountered topics in these clinical settings. Specific attention is given to practical suggestions on how to obtain information, how to generate reasonable differential diagnoses, how to discriminate among diagnoses, and how to succinctly and thoroughly document clinical decisions. The hope is that it will serve as a valuable instruction manual for not only psychiatric interns and medical students, but also psychiatric social workers, nurse practitioners, and physicians in primary care or emergency settings where access to psychiatric consult is not readily available.

In addition to sections that describe the presentations, differential diagnoses, and treatment of each psychiatric disorder, there are a few "special" features scattered throughout *The Guide*. These include **Style Pointer, ED Rounds,** and **Class Notes** sections. The Style Pointer sections provide instruction on how to interview patients presenting with particular issues, with explicit suggestions on how to phrase questions. The ED Rounds sections outline clinical reasoning algorithms in the emergency setting, and the Class Notes sections provide suggestions on how to concisely document your encounters with psychiatric patients, with an emphasis on difficult medical-legal situations in which careful documentation of clinical decision making is especially important.

The Guide is not intended to be exhaustive. For example, the differential diagnoses and treatment of the patient with schizophrenia and a chief complaint of right lower quadrant abdominal pain have been omitted for the sake of brevity. It is assumed that users of *The Guide* have access to facilities that can provide basic medical care. Thus, the discussion of general medical issues is limited to those issues that impact the diagnosis and treatment of psychiatric illness. The reader is referred to the sister manuals in The Washington Manual™ Survival Guide Series for similar discussions of internal medicine, neurology, pediatrics, obstetrics and gynecology, and surgery. It is my hope that *The Guide*, along with the electronic supplement soon to be released, will function as a useful peripheral brain until force of practice renders the information contained within second nature.

Thank you to Carol S. North, M.D., for providing clinical supervision for this project and to Michelle Nichols for assisting with proofreading.

K.S.G.

Key to Abbreviations

A&O	alert and oriented
A/P	assessment and plan
AFF	affect
AIMS	Abnormal Involuntary Movement Scale
ALLG	drug allergies
AST	assets
BAL	blood alcohol level
CC	chief complaint
COG	sensorium and intellect
DAT	dementia of Alzheimer's type
DM	diabetes mellitus
ECT	electroconvulsive therapy
FH	family psychiatric and medical history
FTD	frontotemporal dementia
GAB	general appearance and behavior
HAM-D	Hamilton Depression Scale
HPI	history of present illness
I/J	insight and judgment
ID	identifying information
LBD	Lewy body dementia
MEDS	current medications
MMSE	Mini Mental Status Exam
MSE	mental status exam
N/V	nausea and vomiting
NKDA	no known drug allergies
NMS	neuroleptic malignant syndrome
NOS	not otherwise specified
PMH	past medical history
PTSD	posttraumatic stress disorder
R/O	rule out
ROS	medical review of systems
SH	social and developmental history
SO	source of information
SP	speech
TC	thought content
TP	thought process or flow
VaD	vascular dementia
WNL	within normal limits

So You Want to Be a Psychiatrist...

Keys to Survival

Service is the rent you pay for room on this earth.
—Shirley Chisholm

- **Take care of the patient.** You have been called because someone needs your help. It may be the referring physician. It is most certainly the patient. Assume that you are the best doctor he or she will ever see. Your decisions and actions must be directed in the patient's best interest as though he or she were your parent.

- **If called to see a patient, go see the patient.**

- **Protect yourself from harm at all times.**

- **Collect as much collateral information as possible.**

- **The patient's right to autonomy is subordinate only to his or her safety and the safety of others.**

- **The patient is the one with the illness.** A patient hurling insults is the psychiatric equivalent of a sick infant vomiting. The practice of psychiatry is not "sanitized for your convenience." Expect to be in the line of fire sometimes, and do not take it personally.

- **Know where your help is.** Most people do not know everything. An effective care provider knows when and how to contact colleagues who can provide support. Important numbers a psychiatric house officer must have access to include the service chief or attending physician, medical consult staff, and security.

- **Be kind and respectful to colleagues and staff.**

- **Eat, drink, and sleep when you can.**

- **Enjoy the ride.**

2 Approach to the Psychiatric Patient

Much madness is divinest sense—
To a discerning eye;
Much sense—the starkest madness.

—Emily Dickenson

PSYCHIATRIC DIAGNOSIS

The definitions of mental health and mental illness are hotly debated philosophical topics. Sigmund Freud described mental health as the ability to love and work. Certainly, abstract concepts such as social and occupational adjustment are difficult to define and even more difficult to quantify. Furthermore, social and occupational adjustment can vary from environment to environment. Thus, the psychotic individual, who may function poorly in one culture, may hold a position of respect and power in another. Other definitions have also failed to provide adequate descriptions of illness. If we were to define mental illness as a deviation from measurable norms, our diagnoses would capture those who out-performed, in addition to those who underperformed, test standards. By this definition, genius becomes an illness. Similarly, defining mental illness as a deviation from some utopian ideal, although providing a clear financial advantage for the psychiatric service provider, results in overdiagnosis of the population. Thus, each of these definitions, while of philosophical interest, is of little use in aiding in the diagnosis of brain illnesses that affect behavior.

Because current treatments in psychiatry are most likely providing symptomatic relief rather than treating the underlying pathophysiology of illness, one might ask, "What use is psychiatric diagnosis anyway?" If psychosis is treated with an antipsychotic, whether in the context of depression, mania, schizophrenia, or cocaine intoxication, why spend time trying to discriminate among these causes? Accurate, valid diagnosis is as important in psychiatry as in other areas of medicine. It allows for the prediction of clinical course and treatment outcome, thus facilitating long-term treatment planning for the care of the patient. It also facilitates communication among physicians as well as among researchers investigating the underlying pathophysiology of these complex, multifactoral illnesses.

One proposed method for establishing diagnostic validity in psychiatric illness involves the use of (a) clinical description; (b) lab studies (which have proved difficult to come by for psychiatric illnesses); (c) exclusion criteria to delimit an illness from other disorders that share similar features, or to permit exclusion of borderline cases or doubtful

4

cases; (d) follow-up studies suggesting a common natural course for those included in the diagnosis; and (e) family studies or studies of heritability of a disease [1]. The purpose of this proposal was to establish diagnostic criteria that could be used to reduce the pathophysiologic heterogeneity within any group of patients with a particular diagnosis. This empirical approach was adopted in the *DSM-III* and has been perpetuated throughout the revisions to date, although the vast majority of psychiatric diagnoses listed remain to be validated.

Psychiatric illnesses are currently diagnosed using the *DSM-IV* [2]. For each diagnosis, the *DSM-IV* provides a clinical description with inclusion and exclusion criteria. The patient is assessed along five ostensibly independent "axes" that take into consideration the biological, psychological, and social factors influencing the patient's illness. Axis I includes the major psychiatric and substance use disorders. Personality disorders, mental retardation, and general descriptions of the patient's long-standing coping strategies and interactive styles are reported on Axis II. General medical illnesses are reported on Axis III. Psychosocial stressors and a judgment as to their severity are reported on Axis IV. Finally, a global assessment of the patient's social and occupational function is made on Axis V using a standardized, numeric scale. Although this multiaxial classification system is the convention, keep in mind that it is somewhat arbitrary given that all behavior emanates from the brain, and the brain is prone to illness no different than the pancreas—personality disorders are just as biological as psychosis and diabetes.

Having established criteria for specific illnesses, psychiatric diagnosis is accomplished largely by astute observation of the patient's behavior, considered in conjunction with historic information from the patient and other available sources, a physical and neurologic exam, and occasionally lab findings. The goal of most interventions in the hospital setting is to diagnose and treat emergency psychiatric and medical conditions—those that pose a threat to limb and life—and, once appropriate, to establish a disposition plan whereby the patient can obtain services in an ambulatory setting.

SEEING THE PATIENT

Before attempting to conduct the psychiatric interview consider the following:

- **Who**—Psychiatric evaluations may be requested on patients with specific psychiatric complaints—i.e., those who present with depression, anxiety, psychosis, suicidal ideation or homicidal ideation. In addition, a psychiatrist may be consulted to assess acute changes in mental status, to establish the capacity of patients who are refusing treatment, to aid in the treatment of patients who are hostile or uncooperative, or to help establish whether somatic complaints are a product of psychiatric illness. Often, the psychiatric service is contacted if the patient is not responding well to treatment and the treating service has run out of ideas. Regardless of why you are called your mandate is to *take care of the patient*.

- **When**—*If you are called to see a patient, go see the patient.* Certain occasions require that serial assessments be performed, such as if the patient is intoxicated or delirious.

- **Where**—The interview location should be safe, quiet, and as private as possible without compromising safety. Is there an escape route, or is the patient between you and the door? How is security accessible? Are they in the room? Is there a "panic button"? Who responds if it is pressed, and what is the response time? *Protect yourself from harm at all times.* Never see an agitated patient or one who has been agitated without security present.

- **How**—Evaluating the psychiatric patient involves establishing a well-defined reason for the consultation, collecting information regarding the circumstances that precipitated the consultation, and collecting historic information that will assist in establishing a diagnosis, treatment, and disposition plan. *Collect as much collateral information as possible.* Helpful sources include old records, the consulting treatment team, ancillary care staff, the patient's primary psychiatrist, the patient's family, and, of course, the patient. Ideally it is best to obtain permission from the patient before contacting collateral sources because of the potential for compromising confidentiality. However, in emergent situations it is considered ethical to contact outside sources without the permission of the patient to diagnose and stabilize an emergency psychiatric condition. In some cases, contacting outside sources is mandated—e.g., when the patient has made homicidal statements directed toward a specific individual. When information is obtained from an outside source without consent of the patient, clearly document the reasons in the medical record.

PSYCHIATRIC INTERVIEW

The following elements should be part of every complete psychiatric intake assessment. In addition to containing the information that was obtained, the medical record should contain documentation of what relevant information was not obtained and why.

- **Time and date of the evaluation**

- **Identifying information (ID):** Age, sex, race, referral source.

- **Source of information (SO):** Where did the history come from? Did the patient consent to collateral contacts? If not, why were they contacted without consent? How reliable is the information? If information is judged to be unreliable, what is the basis for this judgment?

- **Chief complaint (CC):** A direct quotation from the patient and the referral source if available.

- **History of present illness (HPI):** What is the sequence of events that led the patient or referral source to seek psychiatric treatment at this particular time? What are the pertinent symptoms or absence of symptoms that suggest a particular diagnosis? Has the patient been previously diagnosed? On what information was the diagnosis based? What treatments has the patient been offered in the past, and were they effective? Does the patient currently have a primary psychiatrist? Are there biological, psychological, or social factors that have complicated treatment or diagnosis such as treatment resistance, noncompliance with treatment, substance abuse or dependence, medical complications, personality disorder, homelessness or poverty, poor social support, etc.? The history of present illness should document any history of mood symptoms (including manic symptoms), psychosis, previous suicide attempts, and hospitalizations for every patient. Substance use history that significantly impacts differential diagnosis should be included here as well. Finally, the HPI should include a statement regarding what treatment or disposition the patient or referral source is expecting.

- **Past medical history (PMH):** Pay special attention to history of head trauma, unexplained loss of consciousness, seizures, or other neurologic illness.

- **Current meds (MEDS):** Names, doses, duration of treatment, recent changes, assessment of compliance.

- **Drug allergies (ALLG):** Medication and allergic response vs. side effect or intolerance.

- **Family psychiatric and medical history (FH):** Is there a history of diagnosed mental illness, "nervous breakdowns," psychiatric contact, substance use, criminal or other antisocial behavior, suicide or suicide attempts? Family medical history, particularly of diabetes, heart disease, obesity, or hyperlipidemia may play a role in treatment selection for some illnesses.

- **Social and developmental history (SH):** Where was the patient born? How far did the patient get in school? Did the patient have behavioral or learning problems in school? Did the patient meet criteria for a conduct disorder or another childhood psychiatric illness? How did the patient relate with friends and family? Is there a history of physical or sexual abuse? How stable have past relationships been? How many times has the patient been married? Does the patient have children? Is there currently a "significant other" in the patient's life? What is the patient's work history? What is the patient's source of income? Where does the patient live and who else is in the house? Is the environment supportive? Is there any history of alcohol, drug, or tobacco use? Are substance use issues currently active?

- **Assets (AST):** From a biological, psychological, and social standpoint, what assets can be used in the treatment and recovery of the patient? Assets may include physical health, stable income or living situation, education, supportive family, good sense of humor, intelligence, insurance, strong therapeutic relationship with a physician, etc.

- **Medical review of systems (ROS)**

- **Complete physical exam (PE):** Includes a neurologic exam.

- **Mental status exam (MSE):** Assess the following elements of mental status:

  - **General appearance and behavior (GAB):** Grooming, psychomotor activity including tremor or dyskinetic movements, eye contact, level of cooperativity.

  - **Speech (SP):** Rate, volume, prosody. Is speech pressured? Is the patient difficult to interrupt? Are there odd word choices or neologism? Clang associations? Word salad? A paucity of speech?

  - **Thought process or flow (TP):** Is it sequential, circumstantial, or tangential? Is there evidence of flight of ideas or loosening of associations? Thought blocking?

  - **Thought content (TC):** Assess for hallucinations (auditory, visual, tactile, olfactory, gustatory); delusions (mood congruent vs. incongruent or bizarre, persecutory, grandiose, erotomanic, thought control, passivity, reference); feeling of helplessness, hopelessness, worthlessness, or guilt; suicidal or homicidal ideation (plan and intent); phobias, obsessions, or compulsions.

  - **Mood:** What does the patient report?

  - **Affect (AFF):** Describe the observed expression of the patient's mood. Is it congruent with the patient's report? Restricted? Full range? Stable vs. labile? Blunted? Flat? Bizarre?

  - **Insight and judgment (I/J):** Does the patient know why a psychiatrist is evaluating him or her? Is the patient seeking treatment? How well can the patient control his or her impulsivity?

  - **Sensorium and intellect (COG):** Level of arousal (alert, attentive vs. inattentive, lethargic, obtunded, stuporous, comatose); orientation (self, place, date, situation); memory (immediate, short term, and long term recall—have the patient repeat three words immediately then test recall at 5 mins); concentration ("Can you say the months of the year forward and backward?"); calculation ("If something cost $1.27 and you paid with a $5 bill, how much change would you get back?"); fund of knowledge ("Name 5 cities; name the last 5 presidents"); reasoning and abstraction (proverb interpretation: "What do people mean when they say 'even monkeys fall from trees/don't cry over spilt milk'?"; similarities and differences:

("How is an apple like an orange? How are they different?"); gross assessment of IQ (below average, average, or above average).

- **Assessment and plan (A/P):** A summary of the case, diagnoses on Axes I–V, and a treatment plan that specifies admission (include indication for admission, precautions to be established and legal status) vs. discharge [include suicide risk assessment, medication changes, follow-up arrangements, and how the patient's safety is going to be managed (e.g., behavioral health hotline, return ED visit, family supervision, or by the patient)].

- **Signature and name printed legibly**

STYLE POINTER: GENERAL INTERVIEW TECHNIQUES

The psychiatric interview cannot be conducted like a "review of systems" interrogation. Patients are often **unwilling or unable** to disclose information regarding their symptoms for various reasons. They may be embarrassed, afraid, too disorganized, or responding to command hallucinations, or they may simply understand the symptoms in a context that differs from how the question was phrased. For example, a patient with schizophrenia may answer "no" to the question "do you ever feel as though people are trying to harm you?" because he *knows* that they are trying to harm him—it's not just a feeling. Thus, the psychiatric interviewer must be attuned to the patient and flexible in the way that he or she phrases questions so as to improve the information yield.

Open-ended and direct questions complement one another in obtaining diagnostic information from the patient. One usually starts with **open-ended questions** that are nonjudgmental and pose no challenge to the patient's belief system. **Directed questions** can then be used to verify the interpretation of open-ended answers. This technique provides the most valid information—the caveat being that patients may avoid discussing uncomfortable material, and thus information can be omitted. A facilitating questioning style that normalizes the patient's experience to the experience of others can be used to elicit endorsements of symptoms that the patient may be reluctant endorse. This approach may lead to over-endorsement of symptoms, and thus it is important to follow up with open-ended questions to verify the endorsement. An example of the use of open-ended, direct, and facilitating questions appears below:

KSG: What brings you into the emergency room? (open-ended)
Patient: I'm depressed.
KSG: How long have you been depressed? (directed)
Patient: I don't know.
KSG: When was the last time you felt good? (directed)
Patient: About two months ago.
KSG: What was going on then? (open-ended)
Patient: I was working. I had plenty of money. My wife and I were getting along.

KSG: What about now? What's changed? (open-ended)

Patient: I lost my job, and no matter how hard I look I'll never find another one.

KSG: It sounds like you're feeling pretty hopeless. (directed to verify interpretation)

Patient: Yep. And I've been so tired lately; I just don't even want to look anymore.

KSG: When people say they are depressed they can mean different things. When you say you're depressed what does that mean? (open-ended)

Patient: Well, for the last two months I haven't been sleeping well, but I'm always in bed. Every time the bills come in I just start crying. I know I could take care of some of them, but I haven't had the energy to write the checks out. That's about it.

KSG: Sometimes when people get depressed they feel like they would be better off dead. Have you ever felt like that? (facilitating)

Patient: Yeah, sometimes.

KSG: Tell me about that. (open-ended verification)

Patient: Well, the other day I was in traffic, and I thought it might just be easier on everyone if I swerved into the embankment and ended it.

KSG: What stopped you? (open-ended)

Patient: Well, I really don't want to die. I love my kids and I want to see them grow up.

Here are some useful interview questions. Remember to be flexible; there are many ways to ask the same question.

- **CC:** This is always an open-ended question. "What brings you into the ED?" "You've been suffering with this problem a long time; why did you decide to come in today?" "What was the straw that broke the camel's back?" "Why do you suppose your family thinks you need to see a psychiatrist?" "Why did the police bring you here and not to jail?" Answers to these kinds of questions help establish the patient's level of insight.

- **HPI:** Again, begin with open-ended questions. "What happens when you (get depressed, manic, hear voices)?" "How have you been spending your time over the past few days?" "Have you ever felt like this before?" "Have you been to see a psychiatrist before?" "What was going on then?" "How were you treated?" "Did it work?" "When was the last time you felt well?" "Can you think of anything that may have triggered these feelings?"

- **TC:** Start with nonjudgmental questions that do not challenge the patient's belief system. Ask regarding the more plausible assertions of the patient first, and then progress to the more bizarre content. Remember to remain neutral. "Is there anyone that you're angry at?" "Why do you suppose (the police, your family, your neighbors, the government) is picking on you?" "How long has this been going on?" "When did you first notice?" "What tipped you off?" "Do you ever feel as though people are spying on you?" "How do they do it?" "Does it seem like they can know your thoughts?" "Do you ever feel like they are putting thoughts in your head?" "Do you ever feel as though someone is communicating with you through the TV or radio?" "Are you a religious person?" "Have you ever had any unusual spiritual experiences?" "Do you ever feel as though you are special or gifted in some way?" "Do you ever hear people talking when no one is in the room?" "What do they say?" "Where do you suppose that comes from?" "Is there anything that you are particularly nervous about?" "How do you keep yourself from getting anxious?" "Do you have any habits or rituals that you perform?"

STANDARDIZED ASSESSMENT TOOLS

Standardized assessment tools exist for almost every psychiatric diagnosis. They are used frequently in research to quantitatively assess patients' symptoms; however, they can be useful in any situation where serial assessment of the patient is desired, specifically if the patient is being assessed over a long period by multiple physicians, such as in a state hospital setting, or if the patient's symptoms fluctuate, such as in delirium. Below are a few of the more commonly used tools (see Appendix G). Other assessment tools may be administered to assess IQ, personality, bizarre thought content, and even malingering.

- **Folstein Mini Mental Status Exam (MMSE)—used to test sensorium and cognition** [3]
- **Hamilton Depression Scale (HAM-D)** [4]
- **Brief Psychiatric Rating Scale (BPRS)** [5,6]
- **Abnormal Involuntary Movement Scale (AIMS)** [7]

LABS AND TESTS

Generally, pursue a medical or neurologic workup whenever you suspect the psychiatric symptoms may have an identifiable, treatable, organic etiology. Consider a more aggressive workup with new-onset illness, acute change in mental status, the presence of constitutional symptoms (e.g., fever), focal or diffuse neurologic signs, or treatment-refractory illness. Labs may also be indicated before starting certain medications. Imaging studies, lumbar puncture, and EEG can also play an important role in the assessment of psychiatric illness. *In this book, the labs and tests that are commonly indicated for workup of each specific clinical situation are listed in the discussion of that situation.*

CLASS NOTES
Psychiatric Assessment

ID: GB is a 28-year-old white male who presents to the ED with his wife.

SO: The following history was obtained from the patient, who appears reliable. His wife was unavailable to provide collateral information although he consented to contacting her.

CC: "My wife said if I didn't get help she was divorcing me."

HPI: This is the first psychiatric contact for this patient, who presents at the demand of his wife after he failed to show up for a job interview that she had arranged for him. The patient reports being in his usual state of mental health until approximately 2 mos ago when he was laid off from his factory job where he had worked the last 7 yrs. The patient reports that afterward he began worrying about finances and was unable to find another job despite multiple interviews. He reported initially having problems with early morning insomnia, and then symptoms progressively worsened, meeting criteria for a major depressive episode. He reports low mood with frequent crying spells. He has not been eating well and has lost 10 lbs. His energy is poor, and he has been lying in bed all day not attending to activities of daily living. As mentioned above, he is not sleeping well. He is unable to concentrate. He endorses feelings of helplessness, hopelessness, worthlessness, and guilt regarding his inability to care for his family. He has had thoughts of death including a fantasy of driving off the road, but he denies any suicidal intent, stating that it would hurt his family too much. He is somewhat ambivalent, however, stating that his wife has not been supportive and perhaps "she deserves to suffer like I have"—a comment on which he would not expound. The patient denies any history of manic symptoms or psychotic symptoms. He has never been previously treated for psychiatric illness. He denies any previous suicide attempts.

His presentation is complicated by a recent increase in his alcohol intake. He reports over the past month using approximately 1 pint of gin daily (he last used 12 hrs ago). He denies previous history of substance dependence, stating that he is usually a "social drinker," having 2–3 mixed drinks 1 weekend each month. He reports several symptom of dependence over the past month including tolerance, loss of control, blackouts, and withdrawal symptoms in the morning. He reports that he missed his interview in part because he was intoxicated.

He comes to the ED with the expectation of receiving inpatient psychiatric care for depression and alcohol use. He reports that his wife is not interested in having him at home until he stops drinking.

PMH: None.

MEDS: None.

ALLG: No known drug allergies (NKDA).

FH: Significant for a father with "alcoholism" and a mother whom he thinks is depressed but has never been treated. His maternal uncle and younger brother both committed suicide. His father has HTN and diabetes. Other family members are alive and well.

SH: The patient was born and raised in St. Louis. He completed high school on schedule with Bs and Cs. He denies any conduct disorder symptoms during childhood. He reports a happy childhood although his father was allegedly verbally abusive when intoxicated. He denies any other abuse. He had a few close friends and married his high school girlfriend when she got pregnant with their first child. They have three healthy children together. After high school, he attended technical school for 1 yr. He has worked for the past 7–8 yrs as a machinist at the same job. He currently owns a home and lives with his wife and children. She provides the only source of income for the household since he lost his job. He denies any legal history other than one arrest for public intoxication after his brother committed suicide 5 yrs ago. He denies illegal drug use. He uses alcohol as outlined above. He smokes 1 pack/day of cigarettes.

ROS: No fever, chills, night sweats, nausea and vomiting (N/V), diarrhea, shortness of breath, chest pain, cough, headache, blurred vision, diplopia, sensory loss, weakness, rash, genitourinary problems.

AST: General health, history of employment, motivated for treatment

PE: Temp: 98.7; heart rate: 110; BP: 160/105; respirations: 16; head: atraumatic normocephalic; eyes: sclera white, pupils equal, round, reactive to light and accommodation, extraocular movements intact, disks: sharp; ears: tympanic membranes clear; neck: supple, full range of motion, no left axis deviation/jugular venous distention; pharynx: nonerythematous, no exudates; chest: clear to auscultation bilaterally; cardiovascular: sinus tach, normal S_1/S_2; abdomen: benign, bowel sounds in all four quadrants; extremities: no clubbing, cyanosis, or edema; skin: diaphoretic.

NEURO: CNs II–XII intact; fine tremor; strength full in all extremities; sensation to temp and position intact; normal station, gait, and gross motor coordination; mildly hyperreflexive throughout.

MSE

- GAB: Cooperative nervous male who appears his age, unwashed, psychomotor retarded, tremulous, poor eye contact

- SP: Decreased volume, rate, and amount

- TP: Sequential

- TC: Feelings of helplessness/hopelessness/worthlessness; thoughts of death but denies overt suicidal ideation (although he made some ominous statements); denies hallucinations, delusions, or homicidal ideation

- Mood: "Pretty bad" "2/10"

- AFF: Dysthymic, restricted

- I/J: Fair

- COG: Alert and oriented $\times$ 3; memory: 3/3 objects at 0 and 5 mins; concentration: can repeat months forward and backward without error although slowly; calculation: $5 - 1.27 = 3.73$; fund of knowledge: able to name five cities and last five presidents; normal proverb interpretation; estimated IQ = average

A/P: 28-yr-old man whose history is consistent with major depressive disorder and alcohol dependence. While not actively suicidal, he has multiple serious risk factors for completed suicide including major depression, alcohol dependence, and recent loss of job, conflict with spouse, and family history of suicide. He also appears to be in active alcohol withdrawal as evidenced by tachycardia, HTN, tremor, and diaphoresis.

Psychiatric Formulation

Axis I:

- Major depressive disorder, single episode, moderate

- Alcohol dependence

Axis II: deferred
Axis III: alcohol withdrawal
Axis IV: marital conflict; loss of job—severe
Axis V: 30–40

I will admit this patient on voluntary status to the dual diagnosis unit. He will be on suicide, elopement, and assault precautions. I will order a urine drug screen, CBC, complete metabolic panel (Sequential Multiple Analysis of 20 chemical constituents), and TSH to assess for any toxic or organic factors that may contribute to this patient's presentation or complicate treatment. The patient's vitals will be monitored for signs of alcohol withdrawal, for which he will receive lorazepam prn. Once medically stable, the patient will attend abstinence groups. I will start sertraline, 50 mg qam, for depression. He will also receive folate, 1 mg qd, and thiamine, 100 mg qd. This case was discussed with the attending physician.

REFERENCES

1. Feigner JP, et al. Diagnostic criteria for use in psychiatric research. *Arch Gen Psychiatry* 1972;26:57–63.
2. The American Psychiatric Association. *Diagnostic and statistical manual of mental disorders,* 4th ed. Washington, DC: American Psychiatric Association, 2000.
3. Folstein MF, Folstein SE, McHugh PR. "Mini-mental state." A practical method for grading the cognitive state of patients for the clinician. *J Psychiatr Res* 1975;12(3):189–198.
4. Hamilton M. Development of a rating scale for primary depressive illness. *Br J Sociol Clin Psychol* 1967;6:278–296.
5. Overall JE, Gorham, DR. The brief psychiatric rating scale. *Psychol Rep* 1962;10:799–812.
6. Woerner MG, Mannuzza S, Kane JM. Anchoring the BPRS: an aid to improved reliability. *Psychopharmacol Bull* 1988;24(1):112–117.
7. Fann WE, et al. Clinical research techniques in tardive dyskinesia. *Am J Psychiatry* 1977;134(7):759–762.

3

Psychiatric Consultation

I would help others, out of a fellow-feeling.
—The Anatomy of Melancholy, *Democritus to the Reader*

COMMON COURTESIES FOR CONSULTING THE PSYCHIATRIC SERVICE

The following practices allow you to call a prompt and effective psychiatry consult, and your efforts will be well appreciated by the psychiatry team.

General

- **Call with a question.** The more specific the question, the more satisfactory the recommendations. For example, rather than say "I have a depressed patient for you to see," formulate the consult as a question—"Can you make treatment/follow-up recommendations? Does the patient have capacity to refuse treatment? Could this presentation be a panic attack?"

- **Have the patient's name, location, and date of birth available.** This information helps the consultant find the patient and obtain old records.

- **Have a brief description of the problem, and what you have done to diagnose or treat the problem thus far.** Include the presenting complaint, treatment course to date (if in the hospital), what behavior precipitated the consult, and as thorough a mental status description as you can provide. Try to do as much as you can on your own before calling the consult. Calling a psychiatric consult because the patient is crying is like calling gastroenterology to perform a rectal exam. All physicians should be able to perform a basic mental status assessment.

- **Ask if there is anything you can do to facilitate the consult.** The psychiatrist may request labs, records, a sitter to supervise the patient, etc.

- **Give the consultant your name and a number** at which you can be reached after the consult is completed.

- **Inform the patient** that a psychiatric consult was called.

On the Floor

- **Assess the patient's mental status thoroughly at intake.** Document level of arousal, orientation, memory, concentration, and language. Nothing is more difficult than assessing a change in mental status when there is no available baseline information. Be sure to document any deviations from baseline on a daily basis—not only obvious, disruptive behavior (agitated, assaultive, naked in the hallway) but also more subtle symptoms that suggest delirium (somnolence, disorientation, incontinence).

- **Assess the patient's drug and alcohol habits at intake.** This will allow you to anticipate and provide prophylaxis for withdrawal syndromes.

- **Avoid stopping the patient's psychiatric medications unless there is a clear medical indication.** If medications are stopped, consult the psychiatric service promptly for additional medication management decisions. Most psychiatric illnesses are more easily managed in remission, so do not wait until the patient decompensates.

- **Use a sitter liberally.** If you are unsure about the safety of a patient, order a staff one-on-one sitter until a psychiatrist can evaluate the patient. Do not allow your judgment to be compromised by staff complaints of "staff shortages." Write the order, call the hospital administrator on duty if needed, and make it happen.

In the Emergency Department

- **Examine the patient before calling psychiatry.** The patient's psychiatric symptoms may very well be a product of a general medical condition or may be secondary to the presenting complaint.

- **Most everyone needs a urine drug screen and a blood alcohol level.** Substances of abuse can precipitate virtually every psychiatric symptom. Even when a patient has a well-documented primary psychiatric illness, substance use can exacerbate underlying conditions and complicate treatment. Furthermore, people frequently do not admit substance use even when directly questioned. Accurate information is essential to diagnose and treat emergency psychiatric conditions.

- **Think "safety."** Do not hesitate to medicate, seclude, restrain, or place with a sitter patients who represent an imminent danger to themselves or others (patients who are assaultive, agitated, pacing in the ED, attempting to elope, or have made a suicide attempt). All patients with suicidal or homicidal ideation should be placed on suicide, assault, and elopement precautions until they are evaluated by psychiatry.

COMMON COURTESIES FOR A PSYCHIATRIC CONSULTATION SERVICE

- **Be kind and respectful to colleagues and staff.** Avoid sarcasm.

- **Write down the name, location, and date of birth of the patient** as well as information on how to contact the consulting service. Verify that the patient has been told that a psychiatric consultation has been called.

- **Try to clarify the nature of the consult request.** Make sure you understand the questions they want answered. Be patient, and help them formulate a question if they are having difficulty.

- **Negotiate the urgency of the consult with the consulting service.** Problems that do not seem urgent to you may be very uncomfortable for them. "I'll be there in 5 minutes/this afternoon/tomorrow. You can keep a sitter in the room until then. Are you comfortable with that?" If the consulting service says the situation is urgent, go see the patient—even if it does not sound urgent. Your over-the-phone assessment of the situation may be inaccurate.

- **Assess the patient completely and answer the consult question,** even if it is not the most critical psychiatric issue that you identify. A thorough assessment of the patient is mandatory. It is not uncommon to be called for recommendations on how to manage a patient's depression when the patient is in fact delirious.

- **Clearly enumerate your recommendations in the chart and leave your contact information.**

- **Contact the consulting service directly regarding recommendations and document the contact.** "These recommendations were discussed with Dr. Whosenheimer."

- **Do not write orders in the chart without the express permission of the consulting service.** When you call with recommendations, say, "If you would like, I can order those medications for you, and you can cosign the order later." Have the unit nurse call the consulting team to obtain verbal verification before orders are executed, thus letting the entire primary treatment team know that at least one member of that team was contacted and agreed with the treatment plan.

- **Before signing off, make sure that any follow-up arrangements are discussed, and offer to help set up appointments.**

TRIAGE AND DISPOSITION PLANNING

It is often the case that the psychiatric consultant is asked to make a decision in the ED or on the floor about the disposition of a patient once he has been medically cleared. The main discrimination to be made is between **admitting the patient to a psychiatric floor** for further stabilization, and **arranging treatment in another setting.** Indeed, assessing the need for inpatient care is one of the most important, yet most difficult, decisions the psychiatric consultant must make.

The decision-making process is further compromised by the fact that admission criteria change in a seemingly arbitrary fashion based on social welfare or insurance company policies that are rarely informed by evidence or outcome studies. Given that the political and economic pressures that shape the criteria set forth by public health facilities and insurance providers may not always work in the patient's best interest, it is important that physicians make it a priority to vanguard the interest of the patient. Observe these principles when determining the disposition of the patient.

- **Accurate diagnosis is critical.**

- **Determine the indicated treatment and treatment setting.** Does the patient need medication? Psychotherapy? Chemical dependency treatment? Is the patient dangerous to self or others?

- **Outline the medically indicated options to the patient along with the risks and benefits of each,** keeping in mind that the patient's right to autonomy is subordinate only to his or her safety and the safety of others.

- **Allow the patient to select** among the medically indicated options.

- **Determine how to allocate resources** to the patient.

- **Carefully document the options that were discussed, and whether the patient has capacity to make an informed decision.** If the patient is discharged, document how follow-up will be arranged and how the patient's safety will be ensured. For example:

  - The risks and benefits of inpatient, partial-day hospital, and outpatient management were discussed and the patient made an informed decision in favor of outpatient management. The patient was given the phone number of the psychiatry clinic and he agreed to call in the morning. His mother felt comfortable supervising his safety and follow-up. The patient and the family were informed that they might return to the ED if symptoms worsen or become intolerable.

INDICATIONS FOR HOSPITALIZATION

As managed care companies set policy to aggressively control the cost of care, the reimbursed indications for hospitalization have become narrowly defined to include, in some cases, only patients who meet the statute criteria for inpatient commitment. A broader and more medically motivated set of criteria are based on the assumption that, in certain situations, hospital care provides a benefit over the outpatient setting in terms of risk management, treatment delivery, or mitigation of suffering. These situations include but are not limited to the following (note that for suicide and assault, *risk* is assessed by the physician and is not necessarily equivalent to *ideation*):

- **Suicide risk** (may also be an indication for involuntary commitment)

- **Assault risk** (may also be an indication for involuntary commitment)
- **Medical instability** (such as with patients who are acutely intoxicated or in withdrawal from alcohol or sedative/hypnotics)
- **Failure of outpatient treatment**
- **Outpatient treatment would result in an unacceptable delay in the delivery of care**
- **New-onset illness**

RELATIVE CONTRAINDICATIONS FOR HOSPITALIZATION

Consider the risks of inpatient care. In some circumstances, it can be argued that inpatient hospitalization is relatively contraindicated because it reinforces maladaptive coping skills and undermines the patient's responsibility for taking a role in his or her treatment. In the following situations hospitalization *may* be a relative contraindication. Keep in mind that risk to the welfare of the patient and others must be assessed with each individual case.

- **Chronic suicidal ideation**
- **Repeated hospitalizations with failure to adhere to after-care plans**
- **Malingering** (there are situations, however, in which admitting a malingering patient is indicated)

CLASS NOTES
Psychiatric Consult

ID: CJ is a 69-year-old African-American male who was admitted to the surgery floor status post hernia repair.

Reason for consult: Psychiatry was called to evaluate and treat possible depression.

SO: The following history was obtained from the patient, who appears unreliable. The patient's son, with the patient's consent, and the chart record, provide reliable information.

CC: Per patient: "I don't know. You'll have to ask them." Per son: "He's not himself."

HPI: The patient, who per his son was treated for a major depressive episode approximately 2 yrs ago after the death of his wife, was functioning at his baseline mental health 4 days before this contact. The patient underwent an elective hernia repair at that time and was admitted to the surgical floor after an uncomplicated surgery. However, he was slow to emerge from anesthesia. Per the consulting service, he has been hypersomnolent and tearful at times over the past 2 days. He will not eat without assistance from the staff or family. No disruptive behavior has been noted in the chart.

The patient's baseline mental status was assessed through information obtained from his son, who reports that he has had some mild cognitive decline. The patient occasionally repeats himself and frequently confuses the names of his grandchildren. He no longer drives due to repeated parking citations for parking the car facing the wrong way on the street in front of his house. His son has been assisting him with his checkbook since the death of the patient's wife. The patient lives alone and does his own grocery shopping and cooking. He lives in a small community and walks to the stores. According to his son, he is fairly active, and before this hospitalization was demonstrating no cognitive or neurovegetative symptoms of depression.

After the death of his wife, the patient suffered what appears to be a single major depressive episode that responded well to citalopram, 20 mg qd. Treatment was complicated by increased use of alcohol that met criteria for alcohol dependence, but the patient denies any use in >1 yr. The patient drank 1–2 12-oz beers almost daily most of his adult life, but was drinking approximately a 12-pack daily for 6 mos before treatment 18 mos ago. The son, who has contact with the patient 4–5 days a week, doubts that he currently uses alcohol. There is no history of psychosis, mania, or suicidal ideation.

On admission, the patient was documented to be alert, oriented, and cooperative—able to provide most of his own history. On exam now, the patient is lethargic but arouses to voice and oriented to self and hospital but not city or date. He is unable to cooperate with much of the mental status exam.

PMH: Type II diabetes, HTN, questionable TIA 5 yrs ago.

MEDS: Before admission: citalopram, 20 mg qd; hydrochlorothiazide, 50 mg qd; glipizide, 10 mg qd; ASA, 325 mg qd; currently these and oxycodone (Percocet), i-ii q6h prn, and lorazepam, 1 mg last hs, for insomnia.

ALLG: NKDA.

FH: Strong history of CVA, HTN, type II DM. No psychiatric history.

SH: The patient was born and raised near Memphis. He dropped out of high school to work on his parents' farm. He is retired and has worked most of his life as a day laborer. He was married for 25 yrs and has 2 children. He used alcohol as outlined above. He smokes 1 pack/day of cigarettes.

ROS: Unreliable.

AST: Supportive family, general health.

PE: See surgical assessment. Of note, the patient is afebrile, vitals are within normal limits (WNL), his abdominal wound appears clean, Foley catheter is in place. Neurologic exam is nonfocal.

LABS: CBC, metabolic panel WNL yesterday.

MSE

- GAB: Lethargic male who appears his age, arouses to voice but needs constant verbal or mild physical prompting to stay awake, psychomotor retarded, no tremor or diaphoresis, poor eye contact.

- SP: Decreased amount, dozes off mid-sentence, naming and repetition intact, understands and follows two-step commands.

- TP: Often tangential.

- TC: Initially believed he was in his kitchen then later said it was the hospital, appears to be responding to visual hallucinations, denies suicidal or homicidal ideation.

- Mood: "Good."

- AFF: Blunted, little range.

- I/J: Poor (does not know where he is or why he is being examined).

- COG: A&O × self only; memory: 2/3 objects at 0 and 0/3 at 5 mins—repeated objects from naming task; concentration: failed to say months forward was perseverant; unable to maintain attention long enough to perform other mental status tasks.

A/P: This is a 69-yr-old man whose history is consistent with major depressive disorder and alcohol dependence, both in remission, and possibly mild dementia. He is now clearly suffering from delirium status post surgery. Possible etiologies for delirium in this patient include, but are not limited to, medications, infection, hypoglycemia, cerebrovascular event (unlikely given nonfocal neurologic exam), or alcohol withdrawal (unlikely given history and presentation).

Psychiatric Formulation

Axis I

- Delirium, NOS (the NOS specification is used until a cause is identified)

- R/O dementia

- Major depressive disorder—in remission

- Alcohol dependence—in remission

Axis II: None
Axis III: Status post surgery, Type II DM, HTN, R/O cerebrovascular disease
Axis IV: Recent surgery
Axis V: 30

Recommendations

1. Discontinue lorazepam and Percocet, as both of these can precipitate delirium in vulnerable individuals. Avoid narcotic analgesics and benzodiazepines.
2. Recommend Tylenol or NSAIDs for analgesia if the patient's pain responds adequately.
3. Because the patient is hallucinating at this time, start a scheduled antipsychotic—haloperidol, 2 mg PO/IM bid.
4. May also use haloperidol, 1–2 mg PO/IM prn agitation; total daily dose not >10 mg.

5. Manage patient's environment with dim lighting, reduced sensory stimulation, frequent reorientation, and family or staff sitter for safety.
6. Would get a fasting serum glucose now to R/O hypoglycemia, and stat basic metabolic panel or Chem 7, CBC, UA with micro, CXR to R/O occult infection and treat as appropriate.
7. We will follow with serial mental status exams.
8. We will reassess for depression and dementia once delirium resolves.
9. Recommendations were discussed with Dr. Cutter.

Common Psychiatric Diagnoses

4

Delirium

Smiles are for youth. For old age come Death's terror and delirium.
—*Philip Larkin*

INTRODUCTION

Delirium is not a single psychiatric illness but rather a set of behavioral symptoms that may arise from multiple toxic and general medical etiologies. Treat delirium as a medical emergency until the underlying etiology is identified and corrected.

DIAGNOSTIC CATEGORIES

Proper diagnosis of delirium involves identifying the syndrome based on its clinical features, then identifying the underlying etiology. The *DSM-IV* specifies diagnostic criteria for five categories of delirium:

- **Delirium due to a general medical condition [specify condition]**
- **Substance intoxication or medication-induced delirium [specify substance]**
- **Substance withdrawal delirium [specify substance]**
- **Delirium due to multiple etiologies**
- **Delirium NOS** (used when clinical features are present but the etiology is unknown)

EPIDEMIOLOGY

It is estimated that 10–15% of surgical and medical patients have delirium [1], and prospective studies indicate the prevalence to be twice as high in hospitalized elderly [2]. Delirium is an indicator of poor prognosis; the mortality rate for hospital patients developing delirium is 20–65% in the hospital [3–5] and is substantially increased in the months after discharge. Risk factors for delirium include

- Advanced age
- Dementia (delirium can be a static feature of dementia)
- Other preexisting CNS pathology (history of stroke, head trauma, mental retardation, seizure disorder)
- Polypharmacy
- Patients in drug withdrawal (benzodiazepines, barbiturates, alcohol)

- Postsurgical setting—particularly postcardiotomy or post–hip fracture repair
- Patients with a multiple illnesses
- Patients with burns
- Patients with AIDS

CLINICAL FEATURES

The core clinical features for delirium include a disturbance of consciousness or awareness of the environment that develops over a short period of time and fluctuates during the course of the day. Delirium may present with symptoms of almost any psychiatric illness. It is differentiated from other diagnoses by the core features, which occur only rarely with primary psychiatric illnesses. Other symptoms may include

- Disorientation (but not always)
- Memory deficits (usually short term and intermediate term)
- Inability to concentrate
- Other cortical deficits (apraxia, acalculia, aphasia, executive function)
- Psychomotor retardation or agitation
- Dysarthria (rare in primary psychiatric illness)
- Disorganized thought process
- Misperceptions and delusions (delusions are usually persecutory, loosely assembled, and the content is local—i.e., the hospital is a prison; bizarre, well-systematized delusions are rare)
- Illusions and hallucinations (vivid hallucinations, visual hallucinations, and tactile hallucinations are suggestive of delirium)
- Affective lability
- Assaultive or suicidal behavior
- Behaviors that interfere with the delivery of treatment, e.g., removing IV lines or Foley catheters
- Sleep disturbances

CAUSES OF DELIRIUM

The assessment of a patient with suspected delirium is incomplete until the diagnosis is made and the underlying etiology has been identified. The diagnosis of delirium is usually established from the history and clinical presentation. A careful history and physical exam along with an appropriate medical workup are pursued to identify the underlying cause with emphasis on ruling out potentially lethal etiologies.

- Infection: central (meningitis, encephalitis) and systemic (pneumonia, urinary tract, HIV, etc.)

- **W**ithdrawal: alcohol, benzodiazepines, and barbiturates

- **A**cute metabolic: acidosis or alkalosis, electrolyte abnormalities, renal or hepatic failure

- **T**oxic: medications (usually benzodiazepines, opioid analgesics, anticonvulsants, anticholinergics, anesthesia), drugs of abuse, metals, pesticides, solvents

- **C**erebrovascular: hemorrhage, infarction

- **H**emodynamic: hypoperfusion of the brain, hypertensive crisis

- **D**eficiencies: Wernicke's encephalopathy, vitamin B_{12}, thiamine, niacin

- **E**ndocrine/**e**lectrical: hypoglycemia, diabetic ketoacidosis, thyroid or adrenal dysfunction/seizure or postictal states

- **A**utoimmune/inflammatory: lupus cerebritis, cerebral vasculitis

- **T**rauma/**t**umor

- **H**ypoxemia: CO poisoning, asphyxiation, pulmonary embolism

ASSESSMENT
HPI

- Collateral informants and a thorough chart review are critical.

- Establish diagnosis based on clinical features.

- Inquire about premorbid mental status with emphasis on predisposing risk factors such as dementia or mental retardation.

- Inquire about previous history of delirium.

- Inquire about substance use history.

- Are symptoms temporally correlated with medicine changes?

- Are symptoms temporally correlated with constitutional symptoms suggesting infection?

PMH

- Is there a history of an ongoing process that could precipitate delirium?

- Cardiac?

- Pulmonary?

- GI hemorrhage?

- Cerebrovascular?

- Seizure?
- Chronic infection (HIV)?
- Endocrinopathy?

MEDS

- Is the patient on any centrally acting substances?
- Are there recent changes?
- Are they temporally correlated with onset of symptoms?

SOC

- A detailed drug and alcohol history is critical.
- Assess premorbid changes in occupational function that may suggest dementia.

PE

- A complete physical and neurologic exam is critical.
- Is the patient febrile?
- Are vitals stable?
- Reactive pupils, nystagmus, scleral icterus?
- Mucosa dry? Hypersalivation?
- Abnormal cardiovascular or pulmonary exam?
- Abdominal tenderness or occult blood in stool?
- Focality on neurologic exam?
- Tremor or rigidity?
- Dysarthria, ataxia, hyperreflexia?

MSE

- Assess mental status frequently to follow course.
- Serial standardized assessment (Mini Mental Status Exam) may be useful.

Lab and Studies

- EEG shows diffuse slowing and may be useful in diagnosing ambiguous cases.
- Use history and physical findings to direct workup.
- Urine drug screen, SMA-20, CBC, and UA with microanalysis are almost always useful.
- Blood gases if indicated by unstable pulse and respiration.

- Blood cultures and CXR if the patient is febrile.
- Neuroimaging studies if physical exam reveals neurologic signs or symptoms, or papilledema.
- Lumbar puncture if meningeal signs are present.

TREATMENT

The most critical focus of the treatment of delirium involves the identification and correction of the underlying cause. Psychiatrists are usually consulted to make recommendations for the management of disruptive behaviors—agitation, psychosis, or sleep disturbance. The following are typical recommendations:

- Use haloperidol (Haldol), 2–10 mg PO/IM bid and q4h prn for agitation (can substitute other antipsychotics such as risperidone (Risperdal), 1–4 mg if the patient will take PO medicine. Avoid low-potency antipsychotics [6].
- Discontinue potentially causal medications. Avoid narcotic analgesics, benzodiazepines (unless the patient is in alcohol, benzodiazepine, or barbiturate withdrawal, the treatment of which is discussed in Chap. 6, Substance-Related Disorders, in the section Alcohol and Sedatives/Hypnotics), sedative-hypnotics, or anticholinergics, as these can exacerbate delirium.
- If an antipsychotic alone is insufficient to maintain sedation, lorazepam (Ativan), 2 mg PO/IM, may be used for severe agitation [7].
- Manage the patient's environment with dim lighting, reduced sensory stimulation, frequent reorientation, and family or staff sitter for safety. May restrain if necessary to prevent injury to the patient or others.
- Follow progress with serial mental status exams.

REFERENCES

1. Wise MG, Gray KF, Seltzer B. Delirium, dementia, and amnestic disorders. In: Hales RE, Yudofsky SC, Talbott JA, eds. *The American Psychiatric Press textbook of psychiatry.* Washington, DC: American Psychiatric Press, 1999;317–362.
2. Francis J, Martin D, Kapoor WN. A prospective study of delirium in hospitalized elderly. *JAMA* 1990;263(8):1097–1101.
3. Guze SB, Cantwell D. The prognosis in "organic brain" syndromes. *Am J Psychiatry* 1964;120:878–881.
4. Rabins PV, Folstein MF. Delirium and dementia: diagnostic criteria and fatality rates. *Br J Psychiatry* 1982;140:149–153.
5. Weddington WW. The mortality of delirium: an underappreciated problem? *Psychosomatics* 1982;23:1232–1235.

6. Breitbart W, et al. A double-blind trial of haloperidol, chlorproma-zine, and lorazepam in the treatment of delirium in hospitalized AIDS patients. *Am J Psychiatry* 1996;153:231–237.
7. Adams F. Emergency intravenous sedation of the delirious, medi-cally ill patient. *J Clin Psychiatry* 1988;49[Suppl 12]:22–26.

Dementia

Memory is the diary that we all carry about with us.

—*Oscar Wilde*

INTRODUCTION

Similar to delirium, the dementias are a set of illnesses that share common behavioral features but have different underlying etiologies. Dementias are defined psychiatrically based on behavioral presentation, and these behavioral syndromes correlate, in general, with specific regional damage to the brain or with particular pathologic findings at autopsy. The correlation is imperfect, however, and there is a great deal of overlap in the histopathologic findings and neuroanatomic involvement of what may be different pathophysiologic entities.

DIAGNOSTIC CATEGORIES

Proper diagnosis of dementia involves identifying the syndrome based on its clinical features, as well as an underlying etiology. The *DSM-IV* specifies diagnostic criteria for six categories of dementia:

- Dementia of Alzheimer's type (DAT)
- Vascular dementia (VaD)
- Dementia due to other medical conditions
- Substance-induced persisting dementia
- Dementia due to multiple etiologies
- Dementia NOS

Other clinically significant dementia syndromes not currently listed in the *DSM* include

- Lewy body dementia (LBD)
- Frontotemporal dementias (FTD)

EPIDEMIOLOGY [1,2]

- 5–10% of individuals >65 yrs old.
- 15–20% of individuals >75 yrs old.
- 25–50% of individuals >85 yrs old.
- Taken together, DAT type and VaD account for 80–90% of all dementias.

- LBDs are probably the second most common dementia.

- Pure cases of neuropathologic VaD are rare with most clinically diagnosed cases having accompanying pathologic findings of DAT at autopsy.

- HIV is the most common cause of dementia in young adults.

CLINICAL FEATURES

Dementia is generally defined as the development of impaired memory and one or more cognitive deficits, including aphasia, apraxia, agnosia, or impaired executive function, that represents a decline from previous function and results in impairment of occupational or social function. The diagnostic criteria for specific dementias vary from one another, however, depending on the predominating clinical features of the dementia.

Other clinical features of dementia may include the following:

- Depression

- Delusions—similar to those seen in delirium, i.e., local, loosely assembled, nonbizarre, with the delusion that people are stealing from them being most common

- Hallucinations—similar to those seen in delirium

- Delirium (may be a static feature of some dementias, particularly LBD)

- Aggression (particularly FTD)

- Personality change (particularly FTD)

- Wandering and other behavioral disturbances

DEMENTIA OF ALZHEIMER'S TYPE [3]

- Histopathologic findings include amyloid deposits in neuritic plaques and neurofibrillary tangles.

- Etiology is heterogeneous including rare mutations of the amyloid precursor protein (chromosome 21) or presenilin proteins (chromosomes 1 and 14), or sporadic cases. Presence of the apolipoprotein E e-4 allele is a risk factor for developing DAT.

- Clinical diagnosis using *DSM-IV* criteria for DAT is confirmed by autopsy in 90% of cases.

VASCULAR DEMENTIA

The vast majority of cases clinically diagnosed have overlapping DAT pathology along with vascular changes. Nonetheless, vascular insults appear to influence the clinical features of dementia, and management of vascular risk factors remains a significant goal of treatment in some patients. The following clinical features help discriminate VaD from DAT [4]. Probable DAT if total points <5; probable VaD if total >6:

- Abrupt onset: 2 points
- Stepwise progression: 1 point
- Fluctuating course: 2 points
- Nocturnal confusion: 1 point
- Relative preservation of personality: 1 point
- Depression: 1 point
- Somatic complaints: 1 point
- Emotional incontinence: 1 point
- History of hypertension: 1 point
- History of strokes: 2 points
- Evidence of atherosclerosis: 1 point
- Focal neurologic symptoms: 2 points
- Focal neurologic signs: 2 points

LEWY BODY DEMENTIA

LBD is characterized histopathologically by intracytoplasmic inclusion bodies similar to those seen in Parkinson's disease (Lewy bodies) widespread throughout the brain. The pathologic findings of LBD overlap with DAT in that as many as 25% of patients with DAT have Lewy bodies, and most patients with LBD have amyloid plaques. In addition to the cognitive deficits common to all dementias, the presentation of LBD is predominated by [5]

- Fluctuation in cognitive impairment similar to that seen with delirium
- Vivid visual and auditory hallucinations occurring early relative to cognitive decline
- Parkinsonian features (bradykinesia, tremor, rigidity, shuffling gait)
- Hypersensitivity to extrapyramidal side effects of neuroleptics

FRONTOTEMPORAL DEMENTIAS

Frontotemporal dementia refers to the behavioral presentation of dementia that is correlated with damage to frontal and temporal lobes. The label includes a heterogeneous group of diseases, because many disease processes that cause dementia can differentially affect these areas. In addition to the cognitive deficits common to all dementias, the behavioral features that suggest FTD include [6]

- Impaired social conduct, manners, or grace
- Lewd language or disinhibited sexual behavior

- Passivity and emotional blunting
- Poor insight
- Poor hygiene
- Hyperorality
- Verbal and behavioral perseveration
- "Frontal release" signs

CAUSES

In addition to DAT and VaD, other causes of dementia include [8]

- LBD
- Pick's disease (FTD)
- Neurodegenerative illnesses (e.g., Parkinson's disease and Huntington's chorea)
- Wilson's disease
- Demyelinating illnesses (e.g., multiple sclerosis and Marchiafava-Bignami disease)
- Trauma, as in dementia pugilistica
- Neoplasm
- Hydrocephalus (dementia, ataxia, and urinary incontinence are the hallmarks of normal pressure hydrocephalus)
- Inflammatory conditions (e.g., sarcoidosis and systemic lupus erythematosus)
- Infection (syphilis, HIV, Lyme disease, Jakob-Creutzfeldt disease, and chronic meningitides)
- Toxic (inhalants, alcohol, anticholinergics, antihypertensives, anticonvulsants, etc.)
- Vitamin deficiencies (vitamin B_{12}, folate)
- Endocrinopathies (thyroid, adrenal)

ASSESSMENT

The diagnosis is made by taking a careful history and mental status exam. Collateral information is critical. The workup should be directed at identifying the underlying etiology or any treatable illnesses that may be exacerbating the patient's cognitive dysfunction.

HPI

- Differential diagnosis includes delirium and depression (pseudodementia).

- Assess time course of symptoms. Dementias are usually chronic and progressive as opposed to the acute, fluctuating course of delirium. Level of consciousness is usually not affected at the time of diagnosis.

- Assess for depressive symptoms. Depressed patients can usually perform adequately on cognitive tasks that are not timed but may appear demented on timed tests due to psychomotor slowing.

PMH

- Cerebrovascular disease suggests possible VaD.

- Cardiovascular disease suggests possible VaD.

- Diabetes is a predisposing risk factor for micro- and macrovascular disease and, thus, VaD.

- Inquire about HTN, a risk factor for VaD.

- Inquire about a history of movement disorder.

- Inquire about a history of delirium.

- Inquire about symptoms of thyroid dysfunction.

- In the young, inquire about HIV status and a history of opportunistic infections.

MEDS

- Many medications can exacerbate underlying cognitive deficits. Most frequent offenders include benzodiazepines, anticholinergics, beta-blockers, and anticonvulsants.

FH

- Inquire about a history of DAT.

- Family history of cerebrovascular or cardiovascular disease is a risk factor for VaD.

- Family history of movement disorder suggests neurodegenerative disease.

SOC

- Use social history to determine the onset and time course of illness.

- Inquire about previous education.

- Inquire about occupational history.

- Inquire about social adjustment focusing on changes from baseline. Does the patient drive? Shop? Prepare meals? Wash laundry? Bathe regularly? Balance a checkbook? Pay bills?

- Inquire about memory lapses (collateral history is useful here). Does the patient repeat himself? Does patient forget important dates (anniversaries, birthdays)? Does patient forget names or call children by the wrong name? Does patient have difficulty finding words? Has patient gotten lost in familiar places? Misplaced objects? Been unable to find his car in the parking lot?

- Inquire about the use of drugs or alcohol.
- Inquire about smoking (risk factor for VaD).
- Inquire about risk factors for HIV in the young.

PE

- A complete neurologic exam is critical.
- Evidence of focal lesion suggests VaD.
- Tremor, dyskinesia, bradykinesia, and ataxia suggest possible neurodegenerative disease.

MSE

- GAB: Patients may be dirty secondary to deteriorating self-care; psychomotor activity may be reduced or there may be evidence of a movement disorder; the patient may appear apathetic or indifferent.
- SP: Patients may search for words (aphasia), and family may complete sentences for the patient.
- TP: May be concrete or may appear circumstantial or tangential as patient confabulates.
- TC: Delusions and hallucinations may be similar to those seen in delirium. Depressive thought content can be a feature of dementia.
- Mood: Patients may reports normal mood or may have difficulty assessing mood. They may be depressed or irritable.
- AFF: May be blunted or indifferent, labile, or euthymic.
- I/J: Patients are often in denial about cognitive deficits.
- COG: Patients may be disoriented and have deficits on memory and concentration tasks, although in the early stages of dementia the MMSE may be normal. Constructional apraxia may be a sensitive test for mild cognitive deficits. Formal cognitive testing may be necessary to assess subtle deficits.

LABS AND STUDIES

- CBC.
- Metabolic panel and electrolytes.
- Thyroid function (TSH).
- Screen for syphilis.

- UA with microanalysis.
- Vitamin B_{12}.
- Folate level.
- Neuroimaging (if neurologic exam or history is equivocal for cerebrovascular disease).
- Lumbar puncture may be indicated to rule in or out some neurologic illnesses or infections.
- HIV status in appropriate risk groups.
- Neuropsychiatric testing can be helpful in the identification and tracking of subtle deficits.

TREATMENT

The approach has four aims:

1. Identify and treat underlying causes of the cognitive deficits:
   - Vitamin replacement for B_{12} or folate deficiencies.
   - Correction of endocrinopathies.
   - Antibiotic treatment for infectious causes.
   - Shunt placement in normal pressure hydrocephalus may be useful.

2. Prophylaxis against symptomatic progression of the illness:
   - Acetylcholinesterase inhibitors delay progression of symptoms in DAT and LBD.
   - Modifying risk factors for cerebrovascular accident such as correcting HTN, controlling diabetes, eliminating tobacco use, and administrating anticoagulants or antiplatelet agents may delay progression of VaD.

3. Optimize the patient in terms of other medical, toxic, or environmental conditions that could exacerbate cognitive deficits:
   - Eliminate alcohol and medication that may impair cognition such as anticholinergic medications, sedatives, and hypnotics.
   - Optimize BP, glucose control, Hgb/Hct, etc.
   - Provide a consistent, structured environment with reinforced daily routine that emphasizes self-sufficiency and completion of activities of daily living.

4. Treat behavioral disturbances associated with dementia, e.g., psychosis, aggression, or depression:
   - Low-dose antipsychotics, preferably those with less anticholinergic activity, can be used to treat aggressive behavior and psy-

chosis associated with dementia. Patients with LBD are extremely vulnerable to extrapyramidal side effects of D_2 antagonists, so low doses of the atypical agents are the treatment of choice.

- Mood stabilizers can be useful in managing mood lability.

- Use antidepressants to treat depression associated with dementia. SSRIs are preferred because of their low side effect profile and low anticholinergic activity. Some data suggest that nortriptyline (Aventyl HCl, Pamelor) may be more effective in poststroke depression, indirectly supporting the role of dual action drugs in the treatment of depression in the context of VaD.

- Cautious adjunctive use of psychostimulants, e.g., methylphenidate (Concerta, Metadate CD, Metadate ER, Methylin, Methylin ER, Ritalin, Ritalin-SR), may improve occupational performance in anergic patients.

EMERGENCY DEPARTMENT ROUNDS: PRESENTATION AND DISPOSITION OF DEMENTIA

Patients with dementia present to the emergency setting for two common reasons. **Acute changes** in mental status may prompt ED visits. These acute changes are usually related to an associated delirium requiring medical workup and treatment. As discussed in the chapter Delirium, delirium can manifest as any of a number of behavioral disruptions including agitation, affective lability, psychosis, and incontinence. The most common underlying etiologies of delirium in such cases are (a) uncomplicated UTI or (b) dehydration. Once identified, the underlying cause can often be corrected in the ED, with IV fluid replacement or antibiotics, for example. In such situations, the disposition decision (discharge vs. admit) is based on the quality of the patient's home care. Usually the patient can be discharged safely to a supervised living environment such as a nursing home. Patients should be admitted for further workup if the underlying cause of an acute change cannot be identified in the ED.

ED visits may also be precipitated when the **chronic progression** of dementia results in a cumulative burden of "nuisance behaviors" that overwhelms the caretaker. These visits are motivated by a desire to control behaviors that are not well tolerated in the patient's current living environment, e.g., assaultive behaviors, wandering behaviors, and urinary or fecal incontinence. In such situations, the patient can be discharged with adjustment in medications (e.g., the addition or titration of antipsychotic medication) if prompt follow-up can be arranged and if the caretaker is comfortable with and capable of supervising the patient's safety, compliance, and follow-up. Otherwise, an admission may be useful in providing the caretaker with respite, allowing time for the adjustment of medications and facilitating the arrangement of enhanced social and medical support for the caretaker (home health, adult daycare, or nursing home placement).

REFERENCES

1. Wise MG, Gray KF, Seltzer B. Delirium, dementia, and amnestic disorders. In: Hales RE, Yudofsky SC, Talbott JA, eds. *The American Psychiatric Press textbook of psychiatry.* Washington, DC: American Psychiatric Press, 1999;317–362.
2. Morris JC. The nosology of dementia. *Neurol Clin* 2000;18(4): 773–788.
3. Cummings JL, et al. Alzheimer's disease: Etiologies, pathophysiology, cognitive reserve, and treatment opportunities. *Neurology* 1998;51[Suppl 1]:S2–S17.
4. Hachinski V. Preventable senility: a call for action against the vascular dementias. *Lancet* 1992;340(8820):645–648.
5. Lapalio LR, Sakla SS. Distinguishing Lewy body dementia. *Hosp Prac* 1998;33(2):93–108.
6. Nearly D, et al. Frontotemporal lobar degeneration: a consensus on clinical diagnostic criteria. *Neurology* 1998;51:1546–1554.

6

Substance-Related Disorders

Drugs bring us to the gates of paradise, then keep us from entering.
—*Mason Cooley*

INTRODUCTION

Substance use disorders are among the most pervasive and costly to society, with 25% of the population fulfilling *DSM* criteria for one or more substance use disorder during the course of their lives [1]. Approximately 60% of these individuals will be dependent on alcohol. In accounting for the social liability incurred from substance use disorders, one must consider costs in the form of lost productivity in the workplace, intoxication-related injuries and accidents, use-related health costs including treatment of the medical sequelae of use and substance use treatment itself, and legal costs. Substance use disorders can mimic virtually every primary psychiatric disorder. This topic and those that follow discuss the presentation of intoxication and withdrawal for various substances and list the related disorders for each.

Abuse and Dependence

Diagnoses of substance abuse or dependence describe pathologic patterns of drug use. *Dependence* refers to an inability to control the intake of a substance ± the presence of physiologic features (e.g., tolerance or withdrawal). In contrast, *abuse* refers to substance use that negatively impacts the social and occupational function of an individual without meeting criteria for dependence [2].

ALCOHOL AND SEDATIVES/HYPNOTICS
General

Alcohol is the most commonly abused drug. Alcohol, benzodiazepines, and barbiturates are cross-tolerant with one another, as they all facilitate neurotransmission via the GABA receptor. Because the intoxication and withdrawal symptoms and the related use disorders are similar, these substances are discussed together [3,4].

Alcohol is consumed orally as commercially available alcoholic beverages of beer, wine, or liquor, but in many "dry" counties in the United States, alcohol is ingested from nonbeverage sources such as mouthwash or cough syrups. Symptoms of intoxication are generally correlated with blood alcohol level (BAL) but vary from individual to individual depending on degree of tolerance. In occasional drinkers, a BAL of 50–75 mg/dL produces euphoria, increased social behavior, and social disinhibition. At a BAL of 100 mg/dL, they become ataxic, dysarthric, and labile, whereas a BAL of 200–300 mg/dL is associated with lethargy and then stupor. Coma and death can occur at a BAL of 400–500 mg/dL. Peak blood levels occur 30–90 mins after ingestion, and alcohol is metabolized at a rate of approximately 30 mg/dL/hr, although this rate depends on tolerance and liver function.

Benzodiazepines and barbiturates are taken orally as pills prescribed by physicians, stolen or obtained by prescription fraud, or purchased from someone who obtained them via such a route. Occasionally, users who have access (commonly health care professionals) will use IV preparations of lorazepam (Ativan), diazepam (Valium, Valrelease), or midazolam (Versed). The duration of action depends on the half-life of the compound used.

Diagnostic Categories for Alcohol and Sedative/Hypnotic Use–Related Disorders

- Dependence

- Abuse

- Intoxication

- Withdrawal

- Intoxication delirium

- Withdrawal delirium

- Induced persisting dementia

- Induced persisting amnestic disorder

- Induced psychotic disorder with delusions or hallucinations

  - May occur during intoxication or withdrawal. Usually self-limited, but should be treated with antipsychotics especially if psychosis is severe or the patient is agitated.

- Induced mood disorder

  - May occur during intoxication or withdrawal, and is usually self-limited. Antidepressant treatment may be warranted if symptoms persist for an extended period during abstinence.

- Induced anxiety disorder

  - May occur during intoxication or withdrawal, and is usually self-limited. Benzodiazepines are useful in the period immediately after substance use ceases. The use of SSRIs may be warranted if symptoms persist for an extended period during abstinence.

- Induced sexual dysfunction

- Induced sleep disorder

- Related disorder NOS

Clinical Features of Intoxication

- Dysarthria
- Ataxia
- Incoordination
- Impaired attention or memory
- Amnesia (blackouts)
- Nystagmus
- Stupor or coma
- Affective lability
- Delirium or hallucinosis may be present

Treatment of Intoxication

- Interrupt use.
- Monitor vital signs hourly for symptoms of withdrawal.
- Gastric lavage with activated charcoal may be useful.
- Support respiration if intoxication is severe.
- Alcohol use may be associated with thiamine, vitamin B_{12}, and folate deficiencies. Thiamine deficiency can lead to Wernicke's encephalopathy, characterized by ataxia, ophthalmoplegia, and confusion. Prolonged encephalopathy can lead to Korsakoff's psychosis, a syndrome of severe anterograde amnesia. Give thiamine, 100–200 mg IV, before glucose administration.
- CBC, serum electrolytes including calcium and magnesium, LFTs, creatinine, BUN, PT, stool guiac, ECG, and serum and urine toxicology aid in assessing risk and anticipating the needs of the patient, should withdrawal symptoms develop.
- IV fluid replacement may be necessary if the patient has been vomiting or is otherwise unable to take PO fluids.
- Place patient in a quiet, controlled environment with reduced sensory stimulation.
- Low-dose, high-potency antipsychotics may be used to control substance-induced psychosis.

Clinical Features of Withdrawal

Withdrawal represents a clinical emergency. Depending on the degree of tolerance, withdrawal symptoms can occur even with substantial blood levels. For example, a patient who is conversant and alert with a BAL of 300 mg/dL may demonstrate significant withdrawal symptoms at 200 mg/dL. Benzodiazepines and barbiturates have withdrawal symptoms similar to those of alcohol, with time courses that vary according to the half-life of the particular substance. In general, short-acting sedatives have a higher risk for abuse, dependence, and withdrawal. Taking an accurate history of substance use allows you to anticipate and provide prophylaxis for withdrawal syndromes. The clinical features are as follows:

- Autonomic instability (diaphoresis, elevated heart rate, elevated BP, anxiety)

- Tremor

- N/V

- Insomnia

- Psychomotor agitation

- Delirium with visual, auditory, or tactile hallucinations

- Generalized tonic-clonic seizures

- Irritability

Treatment of Withdrawal

- Monitor vitals frequently at first (qhr × 12 hrs).

- Use prn benzodiazepines to control autonomic symptoms of withdrawal, anxiety, or insomnia. Depending on tolerance, doses may be very high (>24 mg lorazepam equivalents qd). Patients can be aggressively dosed as long as they are alert (signs of toxicity suggest excessive dosing). Always hold benzodiazepines if the patient is sleeping to avoid respiratory depression. Long-acting agents, such as chlordiazepoxide (Libritabs, Librium, Mitran, Reposans-10, Sereen), are preferred; however, if the patient has hepatic injury, lorazepam, which is cleared by the kidney, can be used instead.

- Consolidate prn dose from the first 24 hrs into a scheduled dose to be tapered over the next 4–5 days.

- Replace vitamin deficiencies with folate, 1 mg PO qd; thiamine, 100 mg PO qd; a multivitamin; and proper nutrition.

- Manage delirium from withdrawal with benzodiazepines as noted above. Low-dose, high-potency antipsychotics may be used adjunctively to treat severe psychotic agitation.

- Seizures can generally be aborted with lorazepam, 2 mg IV; however, sometimes phenytoin (Dilantin, Dilantin-125, Dilantin Infatabs, Dilantin Kapseals, Phenytek) loading is necessary.

Treatment of Dependence

- Treat psychiatric comorbidities (e.g., major depression, anxiety disorders).

- Twelve-step recovery models represent the most successful behavioral approach to abstinence.

- Cognitive behavioral therapy focuses on understanding triggers, thoughts, and feelings associated with use.

- Opiate antagonists, such as naltrexone (ReVia), 25–50 mg PO qd, have been demonstrated to reduce the frequency and severity of relapse for alcohol dependence [5].

- Disulfuram (Antabuse) is effective treatment for alcohol dependence provided compliance can be enforced and the patient is willing [6].

COCAINE, AMPHETAMINE, AND AMPHETAMINE-LIKE DRUGS

General

Cocaine, amphetamine, and amphetamine-like drugs are generally centrally acting sympathomimetics and are either direct agonists of central monoaminergic or serotonergic pathways or act as neurotransmitter reuptake inhibitors. This class includes cocaine, amphetamine, methamphetamine, methylphenidate, and others. As a class, their use-related disorders have similar presentations, so they are discussed together [7,8].

Cocaine in its HCl form is typically "snorted" as a crystaline powder and is absorbed by nasal mucosa; it may also be administered IV. It can also be converted to its freebase form (crack) and smoked. Taken intranasally, cocaine is absorbed over several minutes and has a duration of action of 60–90 mins. Smoking is the most addictive administration route, as there are only a few seconds of delay to onset of action, and the reinforcing effects of the drug rarely last >20 mins. These pharmacokinetics promote a binge pattern of use, wherein users often spend all of their money, then trade personal belongings, then stolen goods and sexual favors for crack.

Amphetamine and methamphetamine (crystal meth, ice, crank) are generally snorted but can be smoked or injected. They are also ingested orally as commercial pharmacologic preparations. Because of the rapid onset of action, smoking and IV routes of administration are highly addictive. The half-life of these drugs is 8–12 hrs. Binging over several days (speed runs) is common.

Diagnostic Categories for Psychostimulant Use–Related Disorders

- Dependence

- Abuse

- Intoxication

- Withdrawal

- Intoxication delirium

- Induced psychotic disorder with delusions or hallucinations

  - May occur during intoxication. Usually self-limited, but should be treated with antipsychotics, especially if psychosis is severe or the patient is agitated.

- Induced mood disorder

  - May occur during intoxication or withdrawal and is usually self-limited. Antidepressant treatment may be warranted if symptoms persist for an extended period during abstinence.

- Induced anxiety disorder

  - May occur during intoxication or withdrawal and is usually self-limited. Benzodiazepines are useful during intoxication. The use of SSRIs may be warranted if symptoms persist for an extended period during abstinence.

- Induced sexual dysfunction

- Induced sleep disorder

- Related disorder NOS

Clinical Features of Intoxication

- Euphoric, expansive, irritable, or labile mood.

- Hypertalkativeness.

- Psychomotor activation including stereotyped movements such as bruxism, lip smacking, or licking.

- Anxiety or hypervigilance.

- Autonomic activation (tachycardia, elevated BP, pupillary dilation, tremor).

- Perspiration.

- Cardiovascular manifestations (e.g., chest pain) may occur.

- N/V.

- Psychosis, including persecutory or grandiose delusions and visual, auditory, or tactile hallucinations ("crank bugs" refer to tactile hallucinations associated with methamphetamine use).

- Delirium and seizures may occur with intoxication.

Treatment of Intoxication

- Interrupt use.

- Obtain ECG and monitor vitals continuously.

- Beta-noradrenergic antagonists (propranolol [Inderal, Inderal LA], 1 mg IV, given slowly) may be used to treat symptomatic HTN or tachycardia.

- Benzodiazepines (lorazepam, 2 mg PO/IM/IV) can be used to reduce anxiety or agitation.

- Give high-potency antipsychotics (haloperidol [Haldol], 2–5 mg PO/IM) if psychotic symptoms are present.

- Acidification of urine facilitates elimination of amphetamine.

- Provide a quiet, safe environment with reduced stimulation.

Clinical Features of Withdrawal

- Occurs shortly after cessation from prolonged use (12 hrs) and can persist for days to months.

- Dysphoric or dysthymic mood.

- Fatigue and sleep changes (usually hypersomnia).

- Psychomotor retardation or activation.

- Vivid or unpleasant dreams (often "crack dreams" are of using).

- Patients may develop suicidal ideation and a profound sense of guilt and hopelessness.

Treatment of Withdrawal

- With the exception of suicide risk, there are no dangerous physiologic sequelae to cocaine or amphetamine withdrawal.

- Mood symptoms are usually mild and self-limited, resolving over days to weeks.

- Desipramine [9] may reduce cocaine craving, although this treatment is controversial.

- Antidepressants are used to treat any persisting or severe mood symptoms.

Treatment of Dependence

- Treat psychiatric comorbidities (e.g., major depression, anxiety disorders).

- Twelve-step recovery models represent the most successful behavioral approach to abstinence.

- Use of antidepressants to manage depressive symptoms that appear during withdrawal may improve quality of life but have little effect on use.

CANNABIS

General

Cannabis, or marijuana, is the most abused illegal substance [10]. The active intoxicants, which include tetrahydrocannabinol, cannabinol, and cannabidiol, are ingested by smoking crushed leaves and flowers of the cannabis plant or by eating or smoking the processed resin (hashish), which may be baked into confections or pastries. The effects of cannabis use are relatively long lasting, with peak plasma levels being reached within 70 mins after smoking or 30–120 mins after oral ingestion. The intoxicating effects usually last 6–8 hrs depending on the amount ingested; however, because cannabinoids are lipophilic; they can be detected in fat or bound to proteins for up to 2–3 wks.

Diagnostic Categories for Cannabis Use–Related Disorders

- Dependence
- Abuse
- Intoxication
- Intoxication delirium
- Induced psychotic disorder with delusions or hallucinations
  - May occur during intoxication. Usually self-limited; treat with anti-psychotics, especially if psychosis is severe or the patient is agitated.
- Induced anxiety disorder
  - May occur during intoxication and is usually self-limited. Benzo-diazepines are useful. The use of SSRIs may be warranted if symptoms persist for an extended period during abstinence.
- Related disorder NOS

Clinical Features of Intoxication

- Euphoria.
- Depersonalization.
- Derealization.
- Sensation of slowed time.
- Impaired coordination.
- Silly or inappropriate affect or laughing.
- Amotivation.
- Conjunctival injection.
- Increased appetite.

- Dry mouth.
- Tachycardia.
- Perceptual disturbances.
- Psychosis, including auditory and visual hallucinations and paranoid delusions (usually that people are watching them or are aware of their use).
- Delirium may occur with intoxication.

Treatment of Intoxication

- Interrupt use.
- Benzodiazepines (lorazepam, 2 mg PO/IM/IV) can be used to reduce anxiety or agitation.
- Give antipsychotics if psychotic symptoms are present.
- Provide a quiet, safe environment with reduced stimulation.

Clinical Features of Withdrawal

Note: No *DSM* category

- Insomnia.
- Nausea.
- Anorexia.
- Irritability and restlessness.
- Yawning.
- Chills.
- Diarrhea.
- Infrequent occurence, only in chronic users of large amounts.
- Symptoms are self-limited and mild, and no pharmacologic management has been demonstrated to be useful.

Treatment of Dependence

- Treat psychiatric comorbidities (e.g., major depression, anxiety disorders).
- Twelve-step recovery models represent the most successful behavioral approach to abstinence.

OPIOIDS
General

Opioids include products derived from the opiate poppy, *Papaver somniferum*, such as morphine and codeine, as well as many synthetic opiate-like drugs, including diacetylmorphine (heroin), and a number of commercially prepared pharmaceutical analgesics. As a class, these drugs are administered via every route available—PO, via intranasal inhalation, by smoking, by injection (IM, SC, or IV), and even as a rectal suppository [11].

Opioids exert their effects via endogenous opiate receptors in the CNS that modulate pain and reward, making them highly addictive. The addictive potential of these drugs largely depends on the potency of the compound used and the route of administration, with IV injection and smoking being the most addictive routes. The pharmacokinetics of opioids vary as well, with withdrawal symptoms emerging hours to days after use is interrupted.

Diagnostic Categories for Opiod Use–Related Disorders

- Dependence

- Abuse

- Intoxication

- Withdrawal

- Intoxication delirium

- Induced psychotic disorder with delusions or hallucinations

  - May occur during intoxication. Usually self-limited, but treat with antipsychotics, especially if psychosis is severe or the patient is agitated.

- Induced mood disorder

  - May occur with prolonged use or during withdrawal and is usually self-limited. Antidepressant treatment may be warranted if symptoms persist for an extended period during abstinence.

- Induced sexual dysfunction

- Induced sleep disorder

- Related disorder NOS

Clinical Features of Intoxication

- Euphoria

- Sedation or sleepiness ("nodding")

- Respiratory depression

- Pupillary constriction (pinpoint pupils)

- Dysarthria

- Impairment of memory or attention

- Perceptual disturbances

- Nausea
- Constipation with decreased bowel sounds
- Reduced sexual desire
- Delirium may occur with intoxication

Treatment of Intoxication

- Interrupt use.
- Monitor vitals continuously. Respiratory depression represents the greatest threat to life.
- Provide respiratory support if necessary.
- If the patient is severely obtunded, naloxone (Narcan), 0.4 mg IV given slowly, may be administered to reverse the effects of intoxication. It may be repeated if no effects are observed. Naloxone can precipitate withdrawal symptoms. Monitor the patient continually as the half-life of most opiates is greater than that of naloxone, and administration may need to be repeated.

Clinical Features of Withdrawal

- Usually develops within hours of cessation of IV usage, or 1–2 days after cessation of oral usage
- Anxiety, irritability
- Insomnia
- Myalgia or muscle cramping
- Headache
- N/V
- Diarrhea or abdominal cramping
- Piloerection ("goose flesh")
- Diaphoresis
- Pupillary dilation
- Lacrimation
- Rhinorrhea
- Yawning
- Fever

Treatment of Withdrawal

Withdrawal is uncomfortable but not life-threatening in healthy individuals. Withdrawal may be managed via three methods [12]:

1. Nonmedical management: involves restricting access to drugs until withdrawal symptoms have run their course.

   • Advantage: discomfort of withdrawal serves as an adverse stimulus to relapse.

   • Disadvantage: poor compliance.

2. Symptomatic management: clonidine (Catapres) (0.1–0.3 mg PO tid–qid prn to control autonomic withdrawal symptoms) and loperimide (Imodium) for diarrhea.

   • Advantage: controls physiologic symptoms of withdrawal without producing euphoria.

   • Disadvantage: does not control psychological symptoms such as craving.

3. Methadone detoxification: start 5–20 mg tid depending on daily use and taper over 4–7 days.

   • Advantage: is cross-tolerant with other opioids; thus, is the most physiologically compatible agent for detoxification.

   • Disadvantage: methadone itself has abuse potential.

Treatment of Dependence [13]

• Treat psychiatric comorbidities (e.g., major depression, anxiety disorders).

• Twelve-step recovery models represent the most successful behavioral approach to abstinence.

• Naltrexone (ReVia), 50 mg PO qd, blocks the rewarding effects of opioids. Effects can be circumvented by using larger quantities or by patient noncompliance.

• Methadone, 60–100 mg PO qd, reduces drug craving and alleviates some of the psychosocial consequences and medical comorbidities of illegal drug use. This maintenance treatment essentially substitutes one addiction for another to facilitate other psychosocial treatments.

• LAAM (levo-alpha-acetylmethadol) is a long-acting opiate agonist (half-life of 92 hrs) that can be used similarly to methadone, with the advantage that it can be dosed every 2–3 days.

• Both methadone and LAAM maintenance therapy can only be prescribed through government-regulated programs.

HALLUCINOGENS
General

The hallucinogen drug class includes *d*-lysergic acid diethylamide (LSD, "acid"), psilocybin, mescaline, and 3,4-methylenedioxymethamphetamine (MDMA, "ecstasy," or "X") [14]. These are characterized by their common ability to alter perception and produce vivid hallucinations. Dissociative phenomena are also common. Hallucinogens produce their effects by modulating serotonergic neurotransmission. The duration of effects varies with dose; however, "trips" of 8–12 hrs are typical, and experiences lasting days are not uncommon.

LSD, a highly potent hallucinogen, was inadvertently discovered by a chemist who absorbed the drug transdermally while attempting to purify the crystals. LSD is usually taken PO in doses of 100–300 μg. It is ingested as a pill or absorbed by the oral mucosa from blotter paper placed under the tongue. LSD can also be administered to unsuspecting victims transdermally by "misting" them with a spray apparatus.

Psilocybin is the psychoactive component in hallucinogenic mushrooms. Mescaline is derived from the peyote cactus. Both mescaline and psilocybin are ingested by eating the plant or fungus, respectively. The duration of action depends on quantity ingested but is typically approximately 4–8 hrs.

MDMA became a popular "club" drug in the mid-1980s, when it was legal for a brief period of time. It has reemerged recently as the drug of choice among college students at all-night dance "raves." MDMA is taken PO as a tablet, and the peak effects usually last 4–6 hrs.

Diagnostic Categories for Hallucinogen Use–Related Disorders

- Dependence

- Abuse

- Intoxication

- Persisting perception disorder (flashbacks)

- Intoxication delirium

- Induced psychotic disorder with delusions or hallucinations

  - May occur during intoxication. Usually self-limited, but treat with antipsychotics, especially if psychosis is severe or the patient is agitated.

- Induced mood disorder

  - Hallucinogens have been shown to be neurotoxic, killing serotonergic cells. Antidepressant treatment may be warranted if mood symptoms persist for an extended period during abstinence.

- Induced anxiety disorder

- Related disorder NOS

Clinical Features of Intoxication

- Visual and auditory illusions and hallucinations.

- Synesthesia: the experience of perceiving sensory input from one modality in another modality (e.g., hearing color or seeing sounds).

- Subjective heightened awareness of sensory input.

- Feelings of depersonalization or derealization.

- Ideas of reference.

- Paranoia or fear of losing one's mind.

- Anxiety or affective lability.

- Autonomic activation (pupillary dilation, tachycardia, sweating, HTN, fever).

- Tremor.

- Blurred vision.

- Incoordination.

- GI symptoms, including N/V, cramping, flatulence, and diarrhea, are common with mescaline and mushrooms.

- MDMA intoxication is more likely to cause heightened sociability, with increased speech, tactile preoccupation, and hypersexuality. Because of the context in which MDMA is used, it is more likely to be associated with the physiologic sequelae of autonomic hyperactivity (e.g., dehydration, cardiovascular crises).

Treatment of Intoxication

- Interrupt use.

- Monitor vitals continuously if unstable.

- Rehydrate if necessary.

- Beta-noradrenergic antagonists (propranolol, 1 mg IV, given slowly) may be used to treat symptomatic HTN or tachycardia.

- Place patient in a quiet environment with decreased stimulation. Familiar, calm friends are useful in reassuring patient that symptoms are related to drug use and will pass.

- Benzodiazepines may be used to treat anxiety or agitation.

- Low-dose antipsychotics may be used adjunctively for sedation and to control psychosis if the patient is agitated or dangerous.

Treatment of Dependence

- Treat psychiatric comorbidities (e.g., major depression, anxiety disorders).

- Twelve-step recovery models represent the most successful behavioral approach to abstinence.

- There is no withdrawal syndrome associated with hallucinogen dependence, nor is pharmacologic management indicated.

PHENCYCLIDINE
General

Phencyclidine (PCP, "angel dust," "water") was developed in the 1950s as an adjunct to anesthesia, producing analgesia and dissociative anesthesia, but was abandoned due to a high incidence of adverse reactions, including confusion and psychosis [14]. PCP became popular after laws were passed regulating the chemicals used to synthesize LSD.

PCP is administered via PO, IV, and intranasal routes, but it is most often smoked with marijuana. Parenteral routes of administration have a quick onset of action (within a few minutes) and a typical duration of action from 4–6 hrs. Psychotic reactions may last weeks, however.

Diagnostic Categories for Phencyclidine Use–Related Disorders

- Dependence

- Abuse

- Intoxication

- Intoxication delirium

- Induced psychotic disorder with delusions or hallucinations

  - May occur during intoxication or persist for weeks beyond discontinuation of use. Use antipsychotics to treat persisting psychosis.

- Induced mood disorder

  - Symptoms are usually self-limited. Antidepressant treatment may be warranted if symptoms persist for an extended period during abstinence.

- Induced anxiety disorder

- Related disorder NOS

Clinical Features of Intoxication

- HTN

- Tachycardia

- Analgesia

- Vertical, horizontal, or rotary nystagmus

- Ataxia

- Dysarthria

- Hypertonia

- Seizure and coma

- Hypersalivation

- Diaphoresis

- Fever

- Auditory hallucinations and delusions

- Affect may be labile or blunted

- Dissociation and inattention

- Odd posturing or repetitive movements

- Catatonia

- Delirium may occur with intoxication

Treatment of Intoxication

- Interrupt use.

- Monitor vitals continuously if unstable.

- Beta-noradrenergic antagonists (propranolol, 1 mg IV, given slowly) may be used to treat symptomatic HTN or tachycardia.

- Place patient in a quiet environment with decreased stimulation. Because of the dissociative nature of intoxication, reasoning with patient or "talking them down" is usually not useful.

- Benzodiazepines may be used to treat anxiety or agitation.

- Antipsychotics may be used adjunctively for sedation and to control psychosis if the patient is agitated or dangerous.

Treatment of Dependence

- Treat psychiatric comorbidities (e.g., major depression, anxiety disorders).

- Twelve-step recovery models represent the most successful behavioral approach to abstinence.

- There is no withdrawal syndrome associated with phencyclidine dependence, nor is pharmacologic management indicated.

INHALANTS [15]
General

Inhalants are a highly varied group of chemicals that function as CNS depressants and produce euphoria when they are vaporized and inhaled. The mechanism of action of these compounds remains unclear; however, the effects can be ascribed partially to their ability to displace O_2 in the lungs and bind Hgb. The use of inhalants as intoxicants is testimony to the lengths people go to get high. They can be divided into three categories: (a) the volatile hydrocarbons such as glues, paints, gasoline, and solvents such as paint thinner; (b) nitrates such as butyl nitrate, amyl nitrate, and NO ("poppers," "rush," "whippets"), which are available in commercial products or used as aerosol propellants in food products; and (c) inhalant anesthetics abused by special populations (health care workers). These drugs are popular because of their ubiquity, lack of regulation, ease of administration, and relatively brief duration of action (seconds to minutes).

Volatile hydrocarbons are general inhaled by one of three methods. Sniffing involves spreading the compound on a piece of wood or cardboard and breathing rapidly and deeply with the nose and mouth approximated to the surface containing the intoxicant. "Huffing" involves breathing the compound through a cloth soaked in the inhalant. "Bagging" refers to a method for concentrating the vaporized fumes by pouring the liquid into a plastic bag, then inhaling and exhaling into the bag.

Nitrates are available in commercial forms in gauze-wrapped glass capsules that are crushed and sniffed, or in screw cap vials. Alternatively, NO is found in tanks or as a propellant in fire extinguishers and food products such as whipped cream.

Diagnostic Categories for Inhalant Use–Related Disorders

- Dependence

- Abuse

- Intoxication

- Intoxication delirium

- Induced persisting dementia

- Induced psychotic disorder with delusions or hallucinations

  - Rarely occurs during intoxication. Usually self-limited, but treat with antipsychotics, especially if psychosis is severe or the patient is agitated.

- Induced mood disorder

  - May occur with chronic use secondary to brain damage. Antidepressant or mood stabilizer treatment may be warranted if symptoms persist for an extended period during abstinence.

- Induced anxiety disorder

- Related disorder NOS

Clinical Features of Intoxication

- Euphoria
- Disorientation
- Memory impairment
- Dizziness
- Confusion
- Headache
- Diplopia
- Dysarthria, ataxia, nystagmus
- Hypotension, bradycardia, arrhythmia
- Injected sclera
- Lacrimation
- Salivation
- Rhinorrhea
- Respiratory wheezing
- Seizures or coma
- N/V
- Hepatotoxicity
- Chemical pneumonitis
- The odor of solvents detected on breath and clothing

Treatment of Intoxication

- Interrupt use.
- Monitor vitals.
- Most symptoms resolve with administration of oxygen.
- CBC, liver enzymes, blood gases, UA and blood toxicology, ECG, and CXR may assist in anticipating the medical sequelae of use.

Treatment of Dependence

- Treat psychiatric comorbidities (e.g., major depression, anxiety disorders).
- Twelve-step recovery models represent the most successful behavioral approach to abstinence.
- There is no withdrawal syndrome associated with inhalant dependence, nor is pharmacologic management indicated.

STYLE POINTER: ASSESSING CHEMICAL DEPENDENCY

Chemical dependency can often be difficult to assess because many patients are not forthcoming with information as a result of fear of stigma or of legal repercussions. Furthermore, many patients minimize the extent or impact of their use. The use of facilitating questions is the approach most likely to yield valid information, as the risk of "false-positive" answers is low (few people exaggerate the extent of their drug use or its impact on their lives). The following example illustrates this technique:

KSG: How old were you when you started to drink?
PT: About 17 years old.
KSG: Do you prefer beer, liquor, or wine?
PT: I drink gin.
KSG: How much gin would you say you drink a day? About 4–5 quarts? (Using exaggeration normalizes experience by allowing the patient to feel he is actually using less than others expect.)
PT: Oh no, I'd never drink that much, are you kidding? Maybe 2 fifths.
or
KSG: So you spend an awful lot of money on cocaine. I bet a person would have to hustle pretty hard to make ends meet. What kinds of things have you done that you might not be so proud of? (Open-ended question can then be followed up with more exploratory questions about prostitution, dealing, stealing, etc.)

When substance use is not part of the presenting complaint, a transition to substance use questions can be made gracefully using other symptoms or complaints to introduce the topic:

KSG: Often people who are as depressed as you are turn to alcohol or drugs to help them cope with the pain. What drugs do you use to help you get through tough times?
or
KSG: Boy, with all of these people trying to listen to your thoughts, it must be pretty stressful. I'll bet you've been tempted to reach for the bottle from time to time.

(First a normalizing statement is followed by a facilitating question that assumes a positive answer.)

A complete history of drug use should include the following elements for each substance:

• When did use start?

• What were the positive consequences of use?

• When did it become problematic in the patient's opinion?

• What quantities are being used?

• Has use increased?

• Has the patient ever tried to quit?

- Were there withdrawal symptoms?

- How long did the patient remain sober?

- What was the patient doing during that time to stay sober?

- What precipitated the relapse?

- Has the patient ever sought formal chemical dependency treatment?

- What have been the medical, legal, social, and occupational consequences of use?

  - Ask about social, occupational, legal, and medical consequences of use: Fighting or arguments? Losing friends? Getting divorced? Interacting with children? Failing to pay bills? Using drugs or alcohol at work? Truancy? Termination secondary to intoxication or use-related absence? Arrests for drug charges? Driving while intoxicated? Public intoxication? Illegal behavior to pay for drugs such as selling, stealing, or prostitution? Assault charges? Health-related consequences? HIV? Hepatitis? Cardiovascular symptoms? Seizures? Withdrawal symptoms? Delirium?

- What is the pattern of use now?

- When did the patient last use?

- What is the relationship between the presenting symptoms and past use?

- Did mood or psychotic symptoms start before, during, or after drug use?

- Assess all patients for risk of dangerous acute withdrawal from alcohol and sedative/hypnotics, as this is life-threatening:

  - When did the patient last use alcohol or sedative/hypnotics?

  - What amount was used?

  - What has been the pattern of use recently?

  - Is there as history of withdrawal seizures?

  - Is there a history of withdrawal delirium?

EMERGENCY DEPARTMENT ROUNDS: DISPOSITION OF THE INTOXICATED PATIENT

Psychiatric consultants are frequently called to the ED to evaluate intoxicated patients who are exhibiting suicidal ideation or psychotic symptoms. The most common intoxicants involved include alcohol and cocaine, although the use of methamphetamine, heroin, and phencyclidine is gaining popularity. The disposition of these patients depends on whether psychosis or suicidal ideation persists after the patient has been adequately detoxified. If the patient is not at risk for a dangerous withdrawal syndrome (as is the case with cocaine and the psychostimulants), you can accomplish this without medication in the ED or in an extended observation unit if one is available. The patients should remain on suicide, assault, and elopement precautions. Adjunctive antipsychotics or benzodiazepines may be administered if the patient is psychotic or agitated. With rest and on regaining sobriety, many patients will recant suicidal ideation when offered chemical dependency treatment. Most large cities have 30-day residential treatment programs that will provide psychosocial stabilization for patients who may have been evicted from their homes by their families or landlords. On completion of "social detox," programs can usually assist the patient in finding community resources to sustain sobriety.

Hospitalization is indicated for patients who

- are at risk for dangerous or uncomfortable withdrawal syndromes (alcohol, sedative-hypnotics, opioids)

- have medical complications from intoxication or withdrawal (such as cocaine-induced ischemia or alcohol withdrawal seizures)

- have persisting substance-induced psychotic symptoms and cannot be discharged to an adequately supervised outpatient environment

- are at risk for completed suicide secondary to comorbid psychosocial conditions that are complicated by substance use

Some states allow patients with chemical dependency to be involuntarily detained for treatment under mental health civil commitment laws; however, data do not support the efficacy of involuntary chemical dependency treatment.

REFERENCES

1. Kessler RC, et al. Lifetime and 12-month prevalence of DSM-III-R psychiatric disorders in the United States: results from the National Comorbidity Survey. *Arch Gen Psychiatry* 1994;51:8–19.
2. The American Psychiatric Association. *Diagnostic and statistical manual of mental disorders,* 4th ed. Washington, DC: American Psychiatric Association, 2000.
3. MacDonald J, Twardon EM, Shaffer HJ. Alcohol. In: Friedman L, et al., eds. *Source book of substance abuse and addiction.* Baltimore: Williams & Wilkins, 1996;109–137.
4. Wiviott SD, Wiviott-Tishler L, Hyman SE. Sedative-hypnotics and anxiolytics. In: Friedman L, et al., eds. *Source book of substance abuse and addiction.* Baltimore: Williams & Wilkins, 1996;203–215.
5. Volpicelli J, et al. Naltrexone in the treatment of alcohol dependence. *Arch Gen Psychiatry* 1992;49:867–880.
6. Wright C, Moore RD. Disulfuram treatment of alcoholism. *Am J Med* 1990;88:647–655.

7. Kerfoot BP, Sakoulas G, Hyman SE. Cocaine. In: Friedman L, et al., eds. *Source book of substance abuse and addiction.* Baltimore: Williams & Wilkins, 1996;157–178.

8. Lit E, et al. Stimulants: amphetamines and caffeine. In: Friedman L, et al., eds. *Source book of substance abuse and addiction.* Baltimore: Williams & Wilkins, 1996;231–242.

9. Carroll KM, et al. Psychotherapy and pharmacotherapy for ambulatory cocaine abusers. *Arch Gen Psychiatry* 1994;51:177–187.

10. Losken A, Maviglia S, Friedman LS. Marijuana. In: Friedman L, et al., eds. *Source book of substance abuse and addiction.* Baltimore: Williams & Wilkins, 1996;179–187.

11. Hirsch D, Paley JE, Renner JA. Opiates. In: Friedman L, et al., eds. *Source book of substance abuse and addiction.* Baltimore: Williams & Wilkins, 1996;189–202.

12. Kleber HD. Opioids: detoxification. In: Galanter M, Kleber HD, eds. *Textbook of substance abuse treatment.* Washington, DC: American Psychiatric Press, 1994.

13. Boyarsky BK, McCance-Katz EF. Improving the quality of substance dependency treatment with pharmacotherapy. *Subst Use Misuse* 2000;35:2095–2125.

14. Brendel D, West H, Hyman SE. Hallucinogens and phencyclidine. In: Friedman L, et al., eds. *Source book of substance abuse and addiction.* Baltimore: Williams & Wilkins, 1996;217–229.

15. Brooks JT, Leung G, Shannon M. Inhalants. In: Friedman L, et al., eds. *Source book of substance abuse and addiction.* Baltimore: Williams & Wilkins, 1996;251–265.

7

Mood Disorders

Manic depression's a frustrating mess.

—*Jimi Hendrix*

INTRODUCTION

Mood disorders are characterized by a primary disturbance of emotion and affect that is associated with a number of neurovegetative symptoms. Like most primary psychiatric disorders, the causes of mood disorders are multifactoral and include genetic predisposition, medical comorbidity, and environmental stressors. The differential diagnosis for mood disorders includes the diagnoses listed below as well as adjustment disorders, personality disorders (particularly cluster B), primary psychotic disorders (such as schizophrenia and schizoaffective disorder), anxiety disorders, and dementia (in the elderly). Always consider and rule out delirium when consulting on the medical or surgical floor for any reason.

DIAGNOSTIC CATEGORIES

There are nine diagnostic categories for mood disorders that can be subdivided into those describing primary unipolar depressive illnesses, those describing bipolar spectrum illnesses, and mood illnesses that occur secondary to other medical conditions and toxins.

- **Major depressive disorder**
- **Dysthymic disorder**
- **Depressive disorder NOS** (used when the patient does not meet complete criteria for major depressive disorder or the etiology is unknown)
- **Bipolar I disorder**
- **Bipolar II disorder**
- **Cyclothymic disorder**
- **Bipolar disorder NOS** (used when the patient does not meet complete criteria for bipolar disorder or the etiology is unknown)
- **Mood disorder due to a general medical condition [specify condition]**
- **Substance-induced mood disorder [specify substance]**
- **Mood disorder NOS**

EPIDEMIOLOGY

Lifetime prevalence of major depressive disorder is approximately 15%, being twice as common in women than men [1].

- Prevalence of bipolar disorder 1–2%; males = females [1].

- 5–15% of adults diagnosed with major depressive disorder eventually meet criteria for bipolar I disorder; approximately one-third meet criteria for bipolar spectrum disorders [2].

- Recurrence rate of major depression after single episode = 50%; 70% after second episode; 90% after third episode [3–5].

- Approximately 10–15% of patients with major depressive or bipolar disorder complete suicide [6].

CLINICAL FEATURES OF THE DEPRESSIVE DISORDERS

This subclass of diagnoses includes major depressive disorder, dysthymic disorder, and depression NOS. The illnesses differ primarily in terms of the severity and chronicity of symptoms; however, they may represent variations of the same underlying pathologic process.

Major Depressive Disorder

Major depressive disorder is a medical illness that is to be distinguished from sadness, disappointment, or grief, which are normal adaptive emotional responses to loss. Unlike these normal emotional responses, patients with major depressive disorder experience perturbations in neurovegetative function (sleep, appetite, motor activity, and energy) and cognition (concentration, executive function, guilt, and suicidal ideation) in addition to low mood or loss of pleasure.

Other clinical features of depression may include

- Anxiety or irritability

- Poor self-care

- Inattention to important life roles (e.g., parenting, work)

- Feelings of helplessness, hopelessness, and worthlessness

- Decreased socialization

- Obsessive rumination on negative themes

- Ideas or delusions of reference (usually mood congruent—e.g., that people are laughing at them or that people are saying negative things about them)

- Delusions of persecution, poverty, or nihilism (usually mood congruent)

- Auditory hallucinations (usually mood congruent, such as a deprecating voice)

- Catatonia
- May be specified as chronic if the symptoms persist >2 yrs

Dysthymic Disorder

Dysthymic disorder is diagnosed when the patient meets partial criteria for a major depressive episode, symptoms persist >2 yrs, and remission of symptoms has never lasted >2 mos at a time. Dysthymic disorder is by definition less severe than depression and is not diagnosed if psychotic symptoms are present. These patients are predisposed to major depressive episodes (a so-called "double depression").

CLINICAL FEATURES OF THE BIPOLAR SPECTRUM DISORDERS

This group of illnesses is characterized by manic symptoms in addition to depressive symptoms. Although the severity and time course differs among diagnoses, these illnesses may represent variations of the same underlying pathologic process. Unipolar mania is not a distinct diagnostic category because although approximately 15% of patients who experience mania will never in the course of their illness meet criteria for a depressive episode, these patients cannot be distinguished from those with bipolar I disorder in terms of other validating criteria (e.g., family history, clinical course) [7,8].

Bipolar I Disorder

Bipolar I disorder is usually characterized by episodic periods of mania (manifested as elevated or irritable mood, grandiosity, decreased need for sleep, racing thoughts, hypertalkativity, distractibility, increased goal-directed behavior, and risk taking) and major depressive episodes. History of a depressive episode is not necessary to diagnose bipolar I disorder. Patients need only meet criteria for one manic episode because epidemiologic data suggest that patients who present with mania will have recurrent episodes of mania and depression. Furthermore, symptoms of depression and mania need not alternate (i.e., manic-depressed-manic-depressed). Patients can have three depressive episodes in a row followed by two manic episodes, for example.

Other clinical features of a manic episode include

- Psychomotor activation
- Increased grooming (excessive jewelry, makeup, flamboyant dress)
- Poor adherence to social boundaries or decreased respect for others' personal space
- Increased playfulness, joking
- Use of clang associations or puns
- Anger and assaultiveness

- Delusions or hallucinations (usually congruent with manic themes such as inflated self-worth, power, wealth, knowledge, or special relationship to a famous person or deity)

- Suicidal behavior

- Catatonia

Bipolar II Disorder

Bipolar II disorder is diagnosed when depressive episodes occur intermittently with manic episodes that are attenuated (hypomanic episodes). Hypomanic episodes differ from manic episodes in that they may be of shorter duration (>4 days vs. >1 wk for a manic episode) and do not cause social or occupational impairment. Episodes that precipitate hospitalization or involve psychosis cannot be diagnosed as hypomanic episodes. History of even one full manic episode prohibits the diagnosis of bipolar II disorder.

Cyclothymic Disorder

Cyclothymic disorder is diagnosed when a patient has had both hypomanic episodes and depressive periods not meeting criteria for a major depressive episode, and these mood symptoms have persisted for 2 yrs without >2 mos of remission at a time. Any history of a manic or major depressive episode precludes the diagnosis of cyclothymic disorder.

CLINICAL FEATURES OF THE SECONDARY MOOD DISORDERS

The secondary mood disorders include mood disorder due to a general medical condition and substance-induced mood disorder. These mood disorders are characterized by a persistent depression or anhedonia, or a persistently elevated, irritable, or expansive mood that occurs in the context of a medical illness or substance associated with such a disturbance of mood.

CAUSES OF MOOD SYMPTOMS [9]

The pathophysiology of the primary mood disorders remains unknown; however, the following general medical conditions are associated with mood disorders:

- Neurologic diseases (neurodegenerative [e.g., Parkinson's and Huntington's], stroke, trauma, dementias, multiple sclerosis, seizure disorder)

- Endocrinopathies (hypo- and hyperthyroidism, diabetes, adrenocortical dysfunction, parathyroid disease)

- Cardiovascular disease

- Sleep apnea and COPD

- Neoplastic (particularly brain tumors or metastases, pancreatic tumors, ACTH-secreting tumors of the lung, adrenal tumors)

- Chronic pain syndromes

- Autoimmune disease (particularly lupus cerebritis, rheumatoid arthritis)

- Metabolic disease or deficiencies (vitamin B_{12}, Wilson's disease, electrolyte disturbances)

The following is a partial list of substances that can cause mood symptoms:

- Substances of abuse (alcohol/sedative-hypnotic, opiate, and psychostimulant use can precipitate depression, but psychostimulants can also induce mania)

- Antidepressants (may induce mania)

- Narcotic analgesics (depression)

- Steroids (mania or depression)

- Anti-parkinsonism agents (mania or depression)

- Antihypertensives (depression, especially reserpine, beta-blockers, and thiazide diurctics)

- Thyroid hormones (mania or depression)

- Antineoplastic agents (usually cause depression)

ASSESSMENT

Initial assessment of mood complaints focuses on accurate diagnosis through careful medical history, psychiatric history, and mental status exam. Triage and disposition of the patient involve an assessment of factors that may complicate treatment or diagnosis, including

- History of alcohol or illicit substance use

- History consistent with comorbid personality disorder

- History of manic symptoms in patients presenting with depression

- Presence of suicidal ideation

- History of previous suicide attempts

- Presence or history of psychosis

- Chronicity of symptoms

- Degree of social support and motivation for treatment

HPI

- In addition to the mood disorders, differential diagnosis includes personality disorder, adjustment disorders, primary psychotic disorders, anxiety disorders, and dementia in the elderly.

- Inquire about the time course of symptoms. Does symptom duration meet criteria for formal diagnosis? Abrupt onset secondary to recent psychosocial stressor suggests adjustment disorder or comorbid personality disorder. Abrupt onset may also coincide with substance use or medicine changes and suggests a substance-induced disorder.

- Inquire about previous episodes. How were they treated? How long did they last? Did they require hospitalization? Did symptoms remit completely? A chronic deteriorating course in a psychotic individual is more suggestive of a primary psychotic disorder. A lifelong history of depressed mood or feelings of emptiness suggests a personality disorder.

- Ask depressed patients about a history of mania. Bipolar illness complicates the treatment of depression because bipolar depression is more difficult to treat and because antidepressants can trigger mania.

- Inquire about current illicit substance and alcohol use. Even if the patient suffers from a primary mood disorder, treatment is ineffective if chemical dependency issues are unresolved.

- Inquire about psychosis. Psychosis is common in bipolar illness and requires adjunct treatment with an antipsychotic. Usually with mood disorders, neurovegetative symptoms and disturbances in mood precede psychotic symptoms. If psychosis precedes mood symptoms, consider the possibility that the patient has a primary psychotic disorder.

- Inquire about suicidal ideation and history of suicide attempts. Chronic, unremitting suicidal ideation suggests a comorbid personality disorder, as do multiple impulsive attempts and self-harming behaviors that are used to modulate affect or manipulate or control others rather than with the intent of suicide. Suicide risk evaluation is discussed separately.

PMH

- Inquire about history of medical illness associated with mood disorders.

MEDS

- Inquire about any recent changes in medications associated with mood symptoms.

FH

- Family history of a mood disorder suggests the same in the patient.

- Family history of a primary psychotic disorder suggests possible psychotic disorder.

- Family history of sociopathy, criminal behavior, etc., or of somatization disorder suggests personality disorder.

- Family history of suicide is a suicide completion risk factor.

- Family history of alcoholism suggests possible substance dependence.

SOC

- Inquire about premorbid function and best level of function.

- Inquire about history suggesting personality disorder, such as legal problems, conduct disorder symptoms, poor job history, discharge from the military.

- Inquire about impulsive lifestyle decisions that may suggest mania—e.g., multiple marriages or affairs, disorganized education or work history, unsound business ventures.

- Inquire about chemical abuse or dependency.

- Inquire about social support structure and current stressors.

PE

- A complete physical and neurologic exam is critical.

- Focus exam on physical findings that suggest illness associated with mood disorders (e.g., cardiovascular, endocrine, neurologic).

MSE

- GAB

  - Depression: Patients may be dirty secondary to deteriorating self-care; psychomotor activity may be reduced or increased with hand wringing, fidgeting, or frank agitation; eye contact may be poor or gaze downcast.

  - Mania: Patients may be overgroomed with excessive makeup or jewelry, odd or flamboyant clothing. They may be psychomotor activated, pacing, unable to sit, intrusive, flirtatious, demanding, or entitled.

- SP

  - Depression: May be quiet, slow, with few words.

  - Mania: May be rapid, loud, difficult to interrupt, pressured, contain clang associations or puns, may persist when the patient is alone.

- TP

  - Depression: May exhibit blocking secondary to poor concentration.

  - Mania: May be tangential or circumstantial, flight of ideas may be present.

- TC
  - Depression: May exhibit feelings of helplessness, hopelessness, worthlessness, guilt, suicidal or homicidal ideation. Hallucinations and delusions usually follow mood-congruent themes such as nihilism, poverty, persecution, or worthlessness.
  - Mania: May feel grandiose or entitled, have delusions or hallucinations centered around mood-congruent themes such as wealth, influence, knowledge, or special relationship to a deity or famous person. Persecutory themes may flow from these as well ("the FBI is trying to kill me because I know how to feed the world"). Suicidal and homicidal ideation occurs in mania. Mood-incongruent or bizarre delusions (e.g., mind control, thought withdrawal) occur with mood disorders but are more typical of primary psychotic disorders.
- Mood
  - Depression: Patients usually report low mood or may have difficulty assessing mood.
  - Mania: Patients report elevated, euphoric mood ("I'm an 11/10, Doc!") or may be angry or irritable.
- AFF
  - Depression: Affect is congruent with mood, may be restricted with diminished range.
  - Mania: May be elevated, expansive, and euphoric with an infectious quality, or may be labile, irritable, and angry.
- I/J
  - Depression: Patients are often in denial, feeling they can "just get over it." They may show great ambivalence regarding treatment but usually respond to gentle challenge.
  - Mania: May feel as though everyone else has the problem. Difficult to engage insight in acutely manic patients, who usually regain insight as mania resolves.
- COG
  - Patients are usually oriented. Both depressed and manic patients can have deficits on memory and concentration tasks, due to inattention. The presence of aphasia, apraxia, or agnosia suggests dementia in patients presenting with mood disorders.

LABS AND STUDIES

All patients should have a primary physician assess their basic medical needs as indicated by exam and history. The following labs and studies represent a minimal assessment for new-onset mood symptoms and serve to provide a baseline health screen before initiating medications:

- CBC

- Metabolic panel and electrolytes

- Thyroid function (TSH)

- Urine drug screen

- Vitamin B_{12}

- Folate level

STYLE POINTER: ASSESSING MOOD DISORDERS

The assessment of depression can be fairly straightforward, as patients often present with depressed mood as their chief complaint. Patients also commonly present with multiple somatic complaints, irritability, fatigue, poor sleep, and failing memory, among others. Patients may be urged to seek help by family members who are concerned about changes in their behavior, emerging psychosis, or suicidal ideation. Finally, patients may seek medical attention for secondary substance dependence or abuse. Assessing patients who present with complaints other than depressed mood can be accomplished by using the chief complaint as a starting point, then gracefully transition to questions about symptoms of depression. For example:

- Why do you suppose you've been drinking so much more lately? With all of the stress in your life, how are your spirits holding up? It sounds like you've been feeling pretty ill. Does it ever affect your mood?

Open-ended questions can help further elicit core symptoms of depressed mood and anhedonia:

- Different people mean different things when they say they are "depressed." What happens to you when you feel depressed? What kinds of things do you do for fun? When was the last time you had fun? When was the last time you felt good?

Often neurovegetative symptoms can be inferred from questions about the patient's day-to-day activities or a change in level of function:

- How are things going at work? Why are you having so much trouble at work lately? Are you having trouble concentrating? How do you spend your time? Why haven't you cleaned the house lately? Are you tired or fatigued? Why are you so tired? Have you been sleeping poorly?

Directed questions can also be used to firmly assess criteria for major depression:

- How has your appetite been? Have you lost/gained weight?

When asking about particularly uncomfortable areas such as **suicide,** asking with a facilitating style helps normalize the patient's experience. Questions about these sensitive topics should begin with the least anxiety-provoking areas and gradually escalate. Try to end with questions that put patients in a more positive frame of mind. Pointing out that the decision to get help is a sign that they are not completely hopeless or helpless may have therapeutic benefit and helps build rapport:

• Sometimes when people are depressed they feel as though "this is how things are and they will never get better" (helpless/hopeless). Have you ever felt that way? Do you ever feel guilty or as though you did something wrong and deserve to feel the way you do? Sometimes when people are depressed their mind plays tricks on them. Have you had any unusual experiences lately where your mind plays tricks on you? For example, they might hear people talking when no one is in the room or feel as though people are watching or talking about them. Have you ever had experiences like that? Sometimes when people are depressed they feel as though they would be better off dead, or like they can't go on. Do you ever feel that way? Have you ever thought of hurting yourself? How did you plan to do it? How far did you get? Did you buy a gun? Did you load it? Put it to your head? What stopped you? What do you have to live for? You are obviously alive right now, so there must be something keeping you going. You're asking for help, so you must have some hope that thing will get better. Hold on to that hope and I'll try to help you feel better again.

Assessing **bipolar illness** is more difficult. Bipolar illness may often present in the manic phase when patients become psychotic, violent, or disruptive. An acutely manic patient may be very psychotic and disorganized, and mania may be difficult to differentiate from schizophrenia. Patients with mania may present to primary care physicians with complaints of insomnia or irritability. It may be difficult to elicit a history of mania from patients presenting with bipolar depression because patients may not have noticed or may not have been disturbed by hypomanic symptoms. Again, use the chief complaint to gracefully transition to questions about mania:

• For depressed patients:

  • Sometimes when people get depressed they will experience periods that are the opposite of depression. Have you ever had a period like that? Have you ever had a period where you feel as though you're on top of the world? You say you're pretty tired right now. Have you ever had periods where you had extra energy, and perhaps didn't need as much sleep? It seems like you're having trouble concentrating right now. Have you ever had a period where your thoughts were moving really fast? It sounds like you're not getting things done very efficiently at work. Have you ever had a period at work where you were especially productive—perhaps taking on more work than you could handle, working more than one job, or putting in late hours?

- For manic patients:

  - You say you haven't slept in two days. Have you needed sleep? Are you tired? How is your energy holding up? You seem irritable. Have you been getting enough sleep? You're talking pretty fast. Are your thoughts moving faster than normal?

Patients may present with frankly delusional claims. Assess **psychosis** in the context of ongoing mood symptoms, focusing on the timing of onset of psychosis in relationship to other mood symptoms. Assess the mood congruency of psychotic themes. When asking about psychotic symptoms, begin with questions that gracefully lead from nonpsychotic material to psychotic material. Remain nonjudgmental using wording that does not challenge the validity of the delusion:

- Are you a religious person? Have you had any unusual spiritual experiences lately? When did you realize you were the reincarnation of Jesus Christ? Have you felt that way all of your life or did it happen just recently? What tipped you off? Was it something you discovered gradually or was there a moment of epiphany? Do you feel as though you have been blessed with special powers or knowledge? Sometimes when people have spiritual experiences like these they will hear the voice of God or the angels or even the devil. Have you heard those kinds of voices? Sometimes they will receive special messages through the TV or radio. Has anything like that happened to you? When all of this started how was your mood? Were you sleeping well then? How about now?

Assess **acutely manic** patients for a history of depression, which aids in confirming the diagnosis of bipolar illness. Acutely manic patients may pathologically deny a history of depression—or any illness for that matter—so look for inconsistencies in the history and follow up on them. These are different ways to get at the same information:

- You look like you're feeling pretty good now, but have you ever had a period where you were sad or blue? Have you ever tried to hurt yourself or to commit suicide? Have you ever been treated for depression? Have you ever been in the hospital because you were depressed? Have you ever had a period where you had less energy, maybe didn't want to get up and do things?

Remember to assess carefully for comorbid disorders that may complicate treatment of mood disorders including substance use and personality disorders. Perform and carefully document a suicide risk assessment on all patients regardless of the presence or absence of suicidal ideation. Suicide risk assessment is discussed more completely in Chap. 12, Suicide Risk Assessment.

TREATMENT OF MOOD DISORDERS

Pharmacologic management of major depressive disorder and bipolar disorder is the standard of care. Offer patients with these diagnoses the option of medication along with a carefully documented discussion of the risks, benefits, side effects, and alternatives.

Bipolar Mania [10]

• Start acutely manic patients on a mood stabilizer and titrate to a therapeutic dose.

• Although the overall efficacy appears about the same, lithium (Cibalith-S, Eskalith, Eskalith CR, Lithane, Lithobid, Lithonate, Lithotabs) may be more effective for euphoric mania, whereas carbamazepine (Atretol, Depitol, Epitol, Tegretol) and divalproex (Depakote, Depakote Sprinkle) may be more effective in mixed or rapid cycling mania.

• Antipsychotics, particularly the novel ones, have been shown effective as adjunctive treatment of acute mania and should be used if the patient is psychotic.

• Some antipsychotics may also be used as monotherapy in acute non-psychotic mania. The effectiveness of antipsychotics in the maintenance phase of mood stabilization is not well studied, however.

• Adjunctive benzodiazepines may be used to treat acute agitation or insomnia.

• Some newer anticonvulsants, particularly lamotrigine (Lamictal), show promise for treating both the manic and depressive phases of bipolar illness.

• Consider discontinuing antidepressants, as these (particularly TCAs) can precipitate manic episodes or induce rapid cycling. Antidepressants may be continued if the patient has a history of refractory depression and manic episodes that are relatively responsive to treatment.

• Consider electroconvulsive therapy (ECT) for refractory cases or when there is a threat of imminent harm to the patient or others.

• Treat comorbid chemical dependency or personality disorders appropriately.

Bipolar Depression [10]

• Place patients on a mood stabilizer along with an antidepressant because antidepressant monotherapy may precipitate mania. Lithium appears more effective in treating bipolar depression than does carbamazepine or divalproex.

• Antidepressants are usually selected based on tolerability, side effect profile, history of response, and family history of response.

- Use as few meds as possible. If the patient fails an adequate trial of one medication, try switching antidepressants. Augmentation strategies include adding an antidepressant from a different class, lithium, thyroid supplementation, psychostimulants, or novel antipsychotics.

- Adjunctive antipsychotics are indicated if the patient is psychotic.

- Adjunctive benzodiazepines may be used to treat acute agitation or insomnia.

- Continue antidepressants for at least 6 mos following remission of symptoms before attempting to taper.

- Continue mood stabilizer treatment indefinitely for relapse prophylaxis.

- Consider ECT for refractory cases, or when there is a threat of imminent harm to the patient or others.

- Treat comorbid chemical dependency or personality disorders appropriately.

Unipolar Depression

- Pharmacologic therapy is similar to that in bipolar illness; however, use of a mood stabilizer is not mandatory.

- Antidepressants are usually selected based on tolerability, side effect profile, history of response, and family history of response.

- SSRIs have been shown to be better tolerated than TCAs in depression after MI [11].

- TCAs may be more effective in treating post-stroke depression; however, risks must be weighed against benefits in this patient population that often has cardiovascular comorbidities [12].

- Use as few meds as possible. If the patient fails an adequate trial of one medication, try switching antidepressants. Augmentation strategies include adding an antidepressant from a different class, lithium, thyroid supplement, psychostimulants, or novel antipsychotics.

- Antipsychotics are indicated adjunctively if the patient is psychotic.

- Adjunctive benzodiazepines may be used to treat acute agitation or insomnia.

- Consider ECT for refractory cases or when there is a threat of imminent harm to the patient or others.

- Treat comorbid chemical dependency or personality disorders appropriately.

- Antidepressants may be carefully discontinued 6–9 mos after remission of depressive symptoms following a single episode. Given the risk of recurrence after two episodes, it is recommended that patients continue to take antidepressants for relapse prophylaxis.

- Cognitive behavioral therapy and interpersonal therapy have documented benefit as adjuncts in the treatment of depression.

CLASS NOTES: DOCUMENTING MOOD DISORDERS

ID: RH is a 37-yr-old white female who presents to the urgent care center at 2:30 A.M.

SO: History was obtained from the patient who appears partially reliable. Collateral information was obtained with the patient's consent from her husband over the telephone.

CC: "I just can't get over this depression."

HPI: The first psychiatric contact for this patient was approximately 10 yrs ago when the patient was started on an antidepressant after the birth of her first child. At the time she reported symptoms that lasted 6 wks and included low mood, poor sleep, poor appetite, psychomotor agitation ("I was unable to sit still"), inability to care for her child due to fatigue and disinterest, and what may have been delusions of poverty ("I was obsessed with the idea that we wouldn't be able to afford to take care of ourselves and the baby, even though my husband had a good job"). The patient was referred to a psychiatrist and was hospitalized briefly "to start medicine" after she revealed to her internist that she was experiencing thoughts of wanting to harm herself and her baby. She was treated with nortriptyline for <1 wk in the hospital then switched to fluoxetine because her symptoms of anxiety and agitation seemed to worsen. She has not seen a psychiatrist in >7 yrs but has continued to take fluoxetine prescribed by her internist.

She now presents with a 3-mo history of depressive symptoms that began when she lost her job. She reports almost continuous feelings of low mood, irritability, psychomotor agitation, decreased sleep, decreased appetite, feelings of failure despite the belief that "I was the most competent worker at that job." Her energy has fluctuated, and at times she is "hyper and can't sit still," although she reports feeling tired most of the time. She denies psychotic symptoms. She denies suicidal ideation at this time, nor any previous attempts. She denies recent alcohol or substance use. She presents now because her symptoms did not respond to an increased dose of fluoxetine, and she was informed today that she could not get an appointment with a psychiatrist for 3 wks. She has been ruminating about her condition all day and came to the urgent care center tonight because she was unable to sleep.

Although she denies a history of a diagnosed manic episode, there is convincing history that she has had at least one manic episode causing impairment in social and occupational function before the current depressive episode. She reports a period of increased productivity at work. She began a second project as a business administrator for a new small business. She was so certain this was going to be successful that she invested all of her savings in the business and worked without pay.

She also purchased an expensive car. She reports not needing as much sleep and working until 4–5 A.M. She would sometimes become very excited about an idea and call her business partners at these late hours. Her husband pointed out to her that she was talking too much about work ("He couldn't shut me up"). During this period she felt "really good." She was discharged from the service of this business venture when, according to her, she requested to borrow back some of the money she had invested to help pay for the car she had purchased.

A number of lifestyle features suggest previous episodes of hypomania. She has been married three times before her current marriage. Each relationship she entered into impulsively after only knowing her partner for a few weeks. None of those marriages lasted >18 mos. Her husband (whom she accuses of being a "tightwad") keeps his money in a separate savings account to which she does not have access, ostensibly because she is frivolous with her money. Her educational and occupational history suggests impulsivity—she has advanced degrees in business administration and social work but has started advanced degree programs in nursing, public health, and romance languages, failing to complete them. She has had multiple jobs, most recently as an inventory manager, but was fired when her personal business venture impaired her performance at work and she yelled at her supervisor.

PMH: None.

MEDS: Fluoxetine, 40 mg qam (increased from 20 mg 2 wks ago).

ALLG: NKDA.

FH: No family history of psychiatric treatment, but her mother "had the blues" after her younger siblings were born. Her father was a real estate speculator who would fluctuate between being very wealthy and being bankrupt, suggesting evidence of bipolar illness. He was affectively labile and "hardly slept." She also reports that he had multiple affairs. She is the oldest of three children. Her siblings are alive and well. Her mother lives alone and has no health problems. Her father died at 67 yrs old of an MI.

SH: The patient was born and raised in Chicago. She completed high school on schedule and was at the top of her class. She denies any conduct disorder symptoms during childhood. She reports a happy childhood without abuse. She became sexually active at the age of 16 yrs old and has had many partners because she says she liked sex. She was very impulsive as a teen and would fall in and out of love easily. This resulted in three impulsive marriages in her early adulthood. She has been married to her current (fourth) husband for approximately 12 yrs and they have one child together. She has had several jobs in the last few years but only recently came on the job market because of her extensive educational history described above. She denies any legal history. She denies illegal drug use but uses alcohol in moderation 2–3 times/mo. She denies tobacco use.

ROS: No fever, chills, night sweats, N/V, diarrhea, shortness of breath, chest pain, cough, headache, blurred vision, diploplia, sensory loss, weakness, rash, genitourinary problems.

AST: General health, above average intelligence, stable relationship and living situation.

PE: Temp: 98.7; heart rate: 72; BP: 130/70; respirations: 16; head: atraumatic normocephalic; eyes: sclera anicteric, pupils equal, round, reactive to light and accommodation, extraocular movements intact, disks sharp; ears: tympanic membranes clear; neck: supple, full range of motion, no left axis deviation/jugular venous distention; pharynx: nonerythematous, no exudates; chest: clear to auscultation bilaterally; cardiovascular: regular rate and rhythm, normal S_1/S_2; abdomen: benign, bowel sounds in all four quadrants; extremities: no clubbing, cyanosis, or edema; skin: clear.

NEURO: CNs II–XII intact; no tremor; strength full in all extremities; sensation to temp and position intact; normal station, gait, and gross motor coordination; reflexes WNL.

LABS: CBC, metabolic panel, electrolytes, TSH WNL; urine toxicology negative.

MSE

- GAB: Cooperative female who appears her age, good grooming with meticulously applied makeup and nail polish, psychomotor slightly agitated, good eye contact, slightly flirtatious

- SP: Normal volume, rate, and amount, although difficult to interrupt

- TP: Sequential usually but circumstantial at times

- TC: Feelings of failure superimposed on some grandiosity regarding her superior working ability, no overt psychosis noted or reported, she denies suicidal or homicidal ideation

- Mood: "Pretty bad but it varies"

- AFF: Labile—dysthymic and crying at times but she will rapidly transition to laughing and joking

- I/J: Fair

- COG: Alert and oriented × 3; memory 3/3 objects at 0 and 5 mins; concentration: can repeat months forward and backward without error; calculation: $5 - 1.27 = 3.73$; fund of knowledge: able to name five cities and last five presidents; normal proverb interpretation; estimated IQ = above average

A/P: This is a 37-yr-old female with a history of major depressive, hypomanic, and manic episodes who has never been treated with a mood stabilizer. Her first depressive episode may have been complicated by psychosis. She now presents after a manic episode with mixed mood symptoms predominated by depressive symptoms.

Psychiatric Formulation:

Axis I: Bipolar I disorder, current episode depressed, moderate

Axis II: Deferred
Axis III: None
Axis IV: Loss of job—moderate
Axis V: 40–50

The patient currently denies suicidal ideation and is requesting out-patient management of her symptoms. She has relatively few risk factors for completion of suicide (no previous attempts, no substance abuse/dependence, no psychosis). She has some protective factors, including a supportive husband. We discussed her revised diagnosis as well as the risks, benefits, and side effects of various treatment alternatives including ECT, and the patient has opted for a therapeutic trial of lithium. I will augment her current dose of fluoxetine with lithium carbonate, 300 mg PO bid (prescription given for #14, no refills), which I will continue for mood stabilization. The patient was also provided with a prescription for zolpidem, 10 mg qhs (#7, no refills) for insomnia. An urgent follow-up appointment was made with me in the clinic tomorrow, and her husband agrees to supervise her compliance with follow-up and medication. The patient understands and agrees with the treatment plan. She knows that she may return to the ED or call me if depressive symptoms worsen, if she develops manic symptoms, or if she develops suicidal or homicidal ideation.

REFERENCES

1. Kessler RC, et al. Lifetime and 12-month prevalence of DSM-III-R psychiatric disorders in the United States: results from the National Comorbidity Survey. *Arch Gen Psychiatry* 1994;51:8–19.
2. Blacker D, Tsuang MT. Contested boundaries of bipolar disorder and the limits of categorical diagnosis in psychiatry. *Am J Psychiatry* 1992;149(11):1473–1483.
3. Frank E, et al. Three-year outcomes for maintenance therapies in recurrent depression. *Arch Gen Psychiatry* 1990;47:1093–1099.
4. Kupfer DJ, et al. Five-year outcome of maintenance therapies in recurrent depression. *Arch Gen Psychiatry* 1992;49:769–773.
5. Thase ME. Relapse and recurrence in unipolar major depression: short-term and long-term approaches. *J Clin Psychiatry* 1990; 51[Suppl 7]:58–59.
6. Guze SB, Robins E. Suicide and primary affective disorders. *Br J Psychiatry* 1970;117:437–438.
7. Nurnberger J, et al. Unipolar mania: a distinct clinical entity? *Am J Psychiatry* 1979;136(11):1420–1423.
8. Pfohl B, Vasquez N, Nasrallah H. Unipolar vs. bipolar mania: a review of 247 patients. *Br J Psychiatry* 1982;141:453–458.
9. Dubovsky SL, Buzan R. Mood disorders. In: Hales RE, Yudofsky SC, Talbott JA, eds. *The American Psychiatric Press textbook of psychiatry*. Washington, DC: American Psychiatric Press, 1999;479–565.

10. Hirschfeld RMA, et al. Practice guideline for the treatment of patients with bipolar disorder. *Am J Psychiatry* 2002;159[Suppl 4]:1–50.
11. Roose SP, et al. Comparison of paroxetine and nortriptyline in depressed patients with ischemic heart disease. *JAMA* 1998;279(4): 287–291.
12. Robinson RG, et al. Nortriptyline versus fluoxetine in the treatment of depression and in short-term recovery after stroke: a placebo-controlled, double-blind study. *Am J Psychiatry* 2000;157(3):351–359.

8 Anxiety Disorders

Anxiety is . . . the uncanny feeling of being afraid of nothing at all.
—William Barrett

INTRODUCTION

Anxiety disorders are a diverse group of illnesses with the common feature that they are characterized by a heightened degree of sympathetic arousal that manifests as nervousness, worry, or panic. Anxiety can be chronic and long lasting (as with generalized anxiety disorder), or it can be discrete and time limited (panic attacks). Anxiety can also be triggered by exposure to provocative stimuli (simple phobias, social phobia) or thoughts (obsessive-compulsive disorder), or they may be a lingering consequence of exposure to extremely noxious stimuli (post-traumatic stress disorder [PTSD]). Finally, anxiety disorders may lead to avoidant behavior that becomes generalized to situations that were not initially provocative (agoraphobia). This topic deals with the diagnosis and treatment of these disorders.

As with other psychiatric illnesses, the differential diagnosis for anxiety disorders is broad and includes medical illnesses (particularly endocrine, cardiovascular, and pulmonary illnesses) as well as primary psychiatric illnesses such as personality disorders (clusters B and C), mood disorders, and psychotic disorders. Because of the overlap between symptoms of anxiety disorders and those of potentially lethal cardiovascular and pulmonary events, a thorough medical workup is mandatory for patients with new-onset anxiety disorders.

DIAGNOSTIC CATEGORIES

- **Panic disorder without agoraphobia**
- **Panic disorder with agoraphobia**
- **Agoraphobia without a history of panic disorder**
- **Specific phobia**
- **Social phobia**
- **Obsessive-compulsive disorder**
- **PTSD**
- **Acute stress disorder**
- **Generalized anxiety disorder**

- **Anxiety disorder due to a general medical condition [specify condition]**
- **Substance-induced anxiety disorder [specify substance]**
- **Anxiety disorder NOS**

EPIDEMIOLOGY [1]
Panic Disorder

- Lifetime prevalence: approximately 3–4%.

- Usual age of onset in early adulthood; rarely occurs after 45 yrs of age. Onset can occur around the time of menopause. Late onset of panic symptoms is strongly suspicious for general medical or toxic etiology.

- 3 times more common in females than males.

- Approximately 50% suffer from agoraphobia.

- Approximately 50% have comorbid depression.

- Symptoms can be chronic or can wax and wane.

Specific Phobia

- Lifetime prevalence is approximately 10%.

- Twice as common in females than in males.

- Age of onset is variable.

Social Phobia

- Associated with shyness in childhood.

- Lifetime prevalence approximately 13%.

- Occurs equally in males and females.

- Usual age of onset in adolescence.

Obsessive-Compulsive Disorder

- Lifetime prevalence 2.5%.

- 75% of onset before age 30 yrs.

- Course may wax and wane with life stress; however, in approximately 15% it is chronic and debilitating.

Generalized Anxiety Disorder

- Lifetime prevalence is 5%.

- Associated with anxiety in childhood or adolescence.

- Females affected twice as frequently as males.

- Often comorbid with symptoms of depression.

Posttraumatic Stress Disorder [2]

- 30–35% prevalence in disaster victims.

- Pretrauma psychiatric diagnosis appears to be a risk factor.

- Normalizing for rates of exposure, women are affected more frequently than men.

- Studies of disaster trauma indicate that 95% of patients meeting category C criteria (avoidance and numbing symptoms) also meet criteria for the full syndrome.

CLINICAL FEATURES

Because panic attacks and agoraphobia are general features of several of the diagnostic categories of anxiety disorders, there are diagnostic criteria that describe these phenomena. Keep in mind that "panic attacks" or "agoraphobia" are not illnesses *per se*. Rather, they are clinical features of other psychiatric syndromes. The duration and frequency of these phenomena and their temporal relationship to provocative stimuli are considered when diagnosing these syndromes.

Panic Attack

A panic attack is a discrete period of anxiety that has an acute onset and a peak symptom intensity occurring within 10 mins. Panic attacks can lead to severe agitation, and patients may appear to be psychotic or become combative as they attempt to escape from provocative stimuli.

Agoraphobia

Agoraphobia is a feature of several anxiety disorders that is characterized by the avoidance of settings in which escape might be difficult in the event of a panic attack. Agoraphobia usually occurs in the context of open spaces such as shopping malls or theaters, at crowded events, or in traffic. Patients may require a familiar person to accompany them in such situations.

Panic Disorder

Panic disorder can be diagnosed with or without agoraphobia when the patient has had recurrent unexpected panic attacks that precipitate concern about having additional attacks, worry about the implication of the attacks, or a change in behavior related to the attacks.

Specific Phobia

Specific phobia refers to an irrational or disproportional fear of a particular situation or stimulus, which predisposes the afflicted patient to anxiety or panic attacks when exposed or when anticipating exposure to that situation or stimulus. Common phobias include fear of animals (e.g,. rodents, spiders, dogs), fear of natural environments (e.g., storms, the ocean, heights), fear of situational stimuli (e.g., flying, elevators, tunnels, traffic), or fear of medical procedures or related exposures (e.g., injury, blood, injections).

Social Phobia

Social phobia refers to a persistent, irrational, or disproportional fear or anxiety that occurs in the context of social performance situations. It is discriminated from agoraphobia in that the anxiety is intimately bound to the social interactions (public speaking, meeting strangers), not the necessarily the inability to escape or unavailability of rescue.

Obsessive-Compulsive Disorder

Obsessive-compulsive disorder is characterized by the presence of involuntary, intrusive, irrational thoughts that provoke anxiety (obsessions), which is alleviated through the performance of repetitive behavioral or mental rituals (compulsions). In general, people with obsessive-compulsive disorder have insight regarding the reality basis of obsessions and compulsions, and those who lack insight appear quite psychotic.

Posttraumatic Stress Disorder

PTSD is a condition that occurs after a person is exposed either through personal involvement, direct eyewitness, or indirectly through the involvement of a loved one to a traumatic event that represents a threat to life or limb. PTSD is characterized by a reexperiencing of the traumatic event, numbing of emotions and/or avoidance of stimuli associated with the trauma, and increased autonomic arousal.

Acute Stress Disorder

Acute stress disorder occurs in the context of life-threatening trauma and is diagnostically similar to PTSD with the exception that the duration is limited to 4 wks and symptoms must occur within 4 wks of the trauma.

Generalized Anxiety Disorder

Generalized anxiety disorder is a condition in which patients suffer excessive worry or anxiety about a number of events or activities, accompanied by psychomotor or neurovegetative symptoms, resulting in an impairment of function. There is a great deal of overlap between symptoms of generalized anxiety disorder and major depression (many patients with major depression have a component of anxiety), making these disorders difficult to differentiate in most cases.

Secondary Anxiety Disorders

The secondary anxiety disorders include those anxiety disorders that can be attributed to a general medical condition or to the effects of medicine, drugs, or alcohol. These drugs or medical conditions can produce symptoms that mimic panic disorder, generalized anxiety disorder, and even obsessive-compulsive disorder.

CAUSES OF ANXIETY

The pathophysiology of the primary anxiety disorders remains unknown; however, the following general medical conditions may mimic anxiety disorders:

- Cardiovascular: angina, MI, hypertensive crisis, mitral valve prolapse, tachyarrhythmias, hypovolemia, shock

- Endocrine: hyperthyroidism, hypothyroidism, hypoglycemia, Cushing's disease, menopause, secreting tumors (e.g., pheochromocytoma), insulinoma, carcinoid

- GI: reflux esophagitis

- Hematologic: anemias

- Postinfectious: pediatric autoimmune neuropsychiatric disorders associated with streptococcal infections (mimics obsessive-compulsive disorder)

- Immunologic: anaphylaxis, SLE

- Metabolic: acidosis, hyperkalemia, hyponatremia, hypocalcemia

- Neurologic: seizures, vertigo, Tourette's disorder

- Pulmonary: asthma, COPD, obstructive sleep apnea, pulmonary embolism, pneumothorax, pneumonia, pulmonary edema

These substances may produce anxiety symptoms:

- Drugs of abuse: alcohol, benzodiazepines, and barbiturates (usually in withdrawal); cocaine and other psychostimulants; caffeine; hallucinogens; inhalants; cannabis

- Pulmonary/ENT medications: theophylline, noradrenergic agonist inhalers such as albuterol, ephedrine and pseudoephedrine, steroids and steroid inhalers

- Psychiatric medications: SSRIs and TCAs; antipsychotics (particularly high potency); anticholinergic medications (benztropine [Cogentin], diphenhydramine [Benadryl, Benylin], trihexyphenidyl [Artane, Artane Sequels, Trihexane, Trihexy-2, Trihexy-5])

- Cardiac medications: epinephrine and other antiarrhythmics; vasopressors (e.g., dobutamine [Dobutrex]), norepinephrine

(Levophed), and phenylephrine (Despec-SF, Neo-Synephrine); antihypertensives

- GI medications: particularly centrally acting antiemetics, e.g., droperidol (Inapsine), prochlorperazine (Compazine, Compazine Spansule), metoclopramide (Reglan), and promethazine (Phenergan)

- Endocrine medications: thyroid supplements, antihyperglycemics, and steroids

- Neurologic medications: amantadine (Symadine, Symmetrel), bromocriptine (Parlodel), levodopa (Dopar, Larodopa)

ASSESSMENT

Given the many dangerous medical conditions that mimic anxiety disorders, a thorough medical evaluation of the presenting complaint is necessary before initiating any psychiatric treatment. Initial assessment of the acutely anxious patient should include a brief history of present illness, a medical history including recent exposures to allergens or toxins, and a complete physical exam. The following initial tests help rule out emergent conditions that cause anxiety:

- Vital signs

- Pulse oxymetry

- Blood gases

- Finger-stick blood glucose

- ECG

- CBC

- Blood electrolytes

- Serum and urine toxicology (to rule out intoxication or dangerous withdrawal syndromes)

After emergent causes of anxiety have been ruled out, a more thorough evaluation can be undertaken. This evaluation is conducted with medical etiologies of anxiety in mind.

HPI

- In addition to the secondary anxiety disorders, the differential diagnosis includes personality disorders, adjustment disorders, primary psychotic disorders, and mood disorders.

- Inquire about the time course of symptoms. Is anxiety chronic or intermittent? Is it related to certain exposures or trauma? Late onset suggests a secondary anxiety disorder.

- Inquire about previous episodes. Do symptoms fluctuate over the years? Have there been associated mood symptoms or psychotic symptoms?

- Inquire about current illicit substance and alcohol use. Even if the patient suffers from a primary anxiety disorder, treatment is ineffective if chemical dependency issues are unresolved.

- Inquire about suicidal ideation and history of suicide attempts. Anxiety disorders carry a risk of suicide completion equivalent to mood disorders.

PMH

- Inquire about history of medical illness associated with anxiety disorders.

MEDS

- Inquire about any recent changes in medications associated with anxiety symptoms.

FH

- Medical conditions that may mimic anxiety disorders may help focus medical workup.

- Family history of a mood or anxiety disorder suggests the same in the patient.

- Family history of a primary psychotic disorder suggests possible psychotic disorder in patients with poor insight.

- Family history of sociopathy, criminal behavior, etc., or of somatization disorder suggests personality disorder.

- Family history of suicide is a suicide completion risk factor.

- Family history of alcoholism suggests possible substance dependence.

SOC

- Inquire about premorbid function and best level of function.

- Inquire about history of trauma.

- Inquire about chemical abuse or dependency.

- Inquire about social support structure and current stressors.

PE

- A complete physical and neurologic exam is critical.

- Exam should focus on physical findings that suggest illness associated with anxiety disorders (e.g., cardiovascular, endocrine, neurologic).

MSE

- GAB: Patients with obsessive-compulsive disorder may be hyper-groomed or unwilling to shake hands because the hospital environment may offer multiple "exposures"; patients with social phobia may appear shy; psychomotor activity may be increased with hand wringing, fidgeting, or frank agitation; eye contact may be poor due to hypervigilance.

- SP: Usually normal

- TP: May exhibit evidence of poor concentration secondary to anxiety or autonomic arousal.

- TC: With the exception of dissociative "flashbacks" in PTSD, which may involve distortions of perception such as illusions, psychotic symptoms are not associated with anxiety disorders. Patients may express feelings of helplessness, hopelessness, worthlessness, guilt, and suicidal ideation. Ask anxious patients about common obsessions or compulsions. Patients with obsessive-compulsive disorder usually have insight with regard to "magical thinking" relating obsessions to compulsions. Lack of insight or thought disorder should prompt a thorough investigation for other psychotic symptoms.

- Mood: Anxious, depressed, or even normal if symptoms are episodic, such as with panic disorder.

- AFF: Patients may be anxious or tearful, or may appear euthymic.

- I/J: Patients with anxiety disorders usually retain insight regarding the fact that there is no harmful threat precipitating symptoms. Acutely anxious patients can use very poor judgment to avoid anxiety-provoking exposures, including attempting suicide.

- COG: Patients are oriented. Acutely anxious patients can have deficits on memory and concentration tasks due to inattention.

LABS AND STUDIES

In addition to labs used in the initial assessment of the acutely anxious patient, the following tests may also be useful in ruling out other medical etiologies:

- Thyroid function (TSH)

- Vitamin B_{12}

- Folate level

- 24-hr urine catecholamine collection to rule out pheochromocytoma

- Sleep studies for sleep apnea

- Pulmonary function tests

- Holter monitor to rule out tachyarrhythmias

- Echocardiogram to rule out valve defects

- Allergen testing

TREATMENT

- With the exception of specific phobia, the mainstay of treatment for anxiety disorders has been the use of antidepressants (particularly SSRIs).

- Treatment usually requires higher doses and longer trials of antidepressants than with major depression.

- Scheduled long-acting, high-potency benzodiazepines, such as clonazepam (Klonopin), are used as adjuncts in the acute phase of treatment and tapered after 2–3 mos of antidepressant therapy at adequate doses.

- Antipsychotics and mood stabilizers can be used adjunctively in the treatment of refractory anxiety disorders, particularly obsessive-compulsive disorder and generalized anxiety disorder.

- Electroconvulsive therapy may be indicated and effective if there are significant mood symptoms.

- The use of high-potency, short-acting benzodiazepines, such as alprazolam (Xanax), is relatively contraindicated in anxiety disorders other than specific phobia, both because of the abuse potential and the complication of rebound anxiety upon withdrawal of the agent.

- The use of high-potency, short-acting benzodiazepines is indicated for simple phobias as needed, when the exposure can be anticipated (e.g., before air travel). Beta-blocking agents, such as propranolol (Inderal, Inderal LA), can be used similarly.

- Various psychotherapies have proven efficacy for anxiety disorders, including flooding, systematic desensitization, relaxation techniques, and cognitive behavioral therapies.

EMERGENCY DEPARTMENT ROUNDS: DISPOSITION OF THE ANXIOUS PATIENT

Disposition of the anxious patient from the ED to the outpatient setting is contingent on the following factors: (a) accurate diagnosis, (b) adequate control of symptoms in the ED, (c) arrangement of prompt follow-up, and (d) determination of minimal suicide risk. If anxiolysis can be accomplished with a fast-acting benzodiazepine (lorazepam [Ativan], 2 mg IM/IV), discharge the patient (with prompt follow-up) on a scheduled high-potency, long-acting benzodiazepine (clonazepam, 0.5 mg bid and 1 mg qhs). Antidepressant medication may be initiated (or the dose optimized if the patient is currently taking an antidepressant) in the ED, particularly if there may be a delay of >1 wk in obtaining follow-up psychiatric care. When prescribing medications from the ED it is prudent to dispense limited amounts (no more than 2 wks) and to document that the risks, benefits, side effects, and alternatives were discussed with the patient.

Inpatient management of anxiety disorders may be indicated (a) to work up new-onset illness; (b) to initiate treatment in particularly severe or treatment-refractory cases in which outpatient management has failed; (c) if the patient is at risk for suicide or deterioration of self-care; (d) if outpatient management would result in an unacceptable delay in the delivery of treatment; or (e) when anxiety symptoms have significant overlap with, or may exacerbate, medical complications (e.g., coexisting cardiopulmonary illnesses).

REFERENCES

1. Kessler RC, et al. Lifetime and 12-month prevalence of DSM-III-R psychiatric disorders in the United States: Results from the National Comorbidity Survey. *Arch Gen Psychiatry* 1994;51:8–19.
2. North CS, et al. Psychiatric disorders among survivors of the Oklahoma City bombing. *JAMA* 1999;282(8):755–762.

Psychotic Disorders

Take care of the sense and the sounds will take care of themselves.
—Alice in Wonderland

INTRODUCTION

Psychosis refers to a disturbance of thought or perception, or a disorganization of behavior. Psychotic symptoms include hallucinations; delusions; breakdown of logical, linear thought; and odd, purposeless, or catatonic behavior. Primary psychotic disorders are a class of illnesses in which psychotic symptoms predominate the syndrome. Psychotic symptoms themselves are neither specific nor pathognomonic of primary psychotic disorders, however, because they may occur during the course of mood disorders (mania or depression), delirium, dementia, and substance intoxication or withdrawal. Some patients with personality disorders (particularly cluster A and borderline personality disorder) may appear psychotic at times, and these diagnoses should be considered in the differential diagnosis of psychosis.

DIAGNOSTIC CATEGORIES

- **Schizophrenia**
  - **Paranoid type**
  - **Disorganized type**
  - **Catatonic type**
  - **Undifferentiated type**
  - **Residual type**
- **Schizophreniform disorder**
- **Schizoaffective disorder**
- **Delusional disorder**
- **Brief psychotic disorder**
- **Shared psychotic disorder**
- **Psychotic disorder due to a general medical condition [specify condition]**
- **Substance-induced psychotic disorder [specify substance]**
- **Psychotic disorder NOS**

EPIDEMIOLOGY [1]
Schizophrenia

- Lifetime prevalence of approximately 1%.

- Onset in late teens or early 20s in males; can be somewhat later in females.

- Characterized by a chronic deteriorating course.

- Suicide rate comparable to depressive illness (approximately 10%).

Schizophreniform Disorder

- Lifetime prevalence of 0.2%.

- Is a provisional diagnosis for most patients who go on to meet duration criteria for schizophrenia.

Schizoaffective Disorder

- Lifetime prevalence of patients meeting strict criteria is low, although it is frequently diagnosed inappropriately.

- Family history reveals schizophrenia in unipolar depressed subtype and bipolar mood disorder in bipolar subtype.

- Risk of suicide is presumed to be similar to mood disorders and schizophrenia.

Delusional Disorder

- Very rare (0.03%).

- Age of onset variable but usually in the 40s.

- Patients are usually refractory to treatment.

Brief Psychotic Disorder

- Also rare.

- High comorbidity with personality disorders, especially cluster B.

CLINICAL FEATURES
Schizophrenia

Schizophrenia was first delineated from other psychiatric illnesses in the early 1900s by **Emil Kraepelin,** who differentiated schizophrenia, then referred to as "dementia praecox," from bipolar illness and other dementias on the basis of its natural clinical history [2]. Subsequently, **Eugen Bleuler** successfully advocated the use of the word *schizophrenia* to describe the illness, as careful clinical observation had led him to the conclusion that the underlying cognitive impairment was a splitting or loosening of associations. Bleuler's clinical observations regarding the presentation of schizophrenia are often taught as the **Four A's** [3]:

- **A**ssociations—as in loosening of association
- **A**ffect—flattening
- **A**utism—refers to bizarre or magical thinking
- **A**mbivalence—or indecisiveness

Finally, the current criteria used to diagnose schizophrenia were influenced by the work of **Kurt Schneider,** who provided descriptions of symptoms that he believed typified the psychosis of schizophrenia. These so-called **first-rank symptoms** focused more on cross-sectional presentation and included

- Audible thoughts
- Auditory hallucinations of two individuals arguing or conversing
- Hallucinated voices commenting on the patient's actions
- Delusions of thought broadcasting
- Delusions of thought withdrawal
- Delusions of thought insertion
- Delusions of somatic passivity (that someone is controlling their actions)
- Somatic hallucinations attributed to outside influences (aliens, poisons)
- Delusions of emotional passivity
- Delusions of reference

These ideas of Kraepelin, Bleuler, and Schneider were incorporated into the modern diagnostic criteria. The syndrome can be further classified according to which symptoms predominate the presentation.

- **Paranoid type** is characterized by predominately positive symptoms (hallucinations and delusions) without prominent disorganization, flattening of affect, or catatonic behavior.
- **Disorganized type,** previously described as hebephrenic, is characterized by prominent thought disorder, disorganization of behavior or speech, and flattening of affect.
- **Catatonic type** is a form of schizophrenia that is dominated by catatonic symptoms. Keep in mind that catatonia may occur with other psychiatric and general medical disorders and is not pathognomonic for schizophrenia.
- **Undifferentiated type** is diagnosed when the patient meets criteria for schizophrenia but does not meet criteria for paranoid, disorganized, or catatonic types.

- Finally, patients who do not meet criteria for one of the other types, who continue to have negative symptoms (i.e., flat affect, alogia, or avolition) and attenuated forms of at least two other criteria A symptoms of schizophrenia, can be diagnosed as **residual type.**

Keep in mind that the subtyping of schizophrenia serves a descriptive purpose only. There are currently little data to support the assertion that these subtypes represent separate illnesses with etiologies distinct from one another.

Schizophreniform Disorder

Schizophreniform disorder is diagnosed if patients meet criteria A, D, and E of schizophrenia for an episode that lasts >1 mo but <6 mos. Good prognostic features of schizophreniform disorder include good premorbid function, acute onset, perplexity or confusion regarding symptoms, and preserved affect.

Schizoaffective Disorder

Schizoaffective disorder is an imprecise and heterogeneous diagnosis used to describe patients who have a psychiatric presentation or longitudinal course that meets criteria for both schizophrenia and a mood disorder (either bipolar or major depressive disorder). It is distinct from a mood episode with psychotic features in that psychotic symptoms persist in the absence of prominent mood symptoms.

Delusional Disorder

Delusional disorder is a rare condition in which the patient has a single, nonbizarre delusion (i.e., involving a situation that could occur in real life) lasting >1 mo, and the patient never met criteria A for schizophrenia. Apart from the impact of the delusion, the patient's behavior cannot be bizarre or significantly impaired in other ways. Typical delusions include erotomanic delusions, jealous delusions, persecutory delusions, delusions of contamination or illness, or grandiose delusions.

Brief Psychotic Disorder

Brief psychotic disorder is diagnosed when symptoms occur with an acute onset and last >1 day but <1 mo. This diagnosis is not used if psychosis is secondary to drugs or a medical condition, or if symptoms are not better accounted for by a diagnosis of schizophrenia or mood disorder. The diagnosis can be further categorized according to whether the onset occurs with or without a precipitating stressor or in a postpartum setting.

Shared Psychotic Disorder (*Folie à Deux*)

Shared psychotic disorder is descriptive of a phenomenon that rarely occurs outside the context of other diagnosable psychiatric illnesses. It is diagnosed when a patient acquires a delusion that is similar in content to an established delusion exhibited by another individual with whom they are in close contact. Patients are excluded if the psychosis can be better accounted for by another diagnosis (e.g., schizophrenia, mood disorder). These patients are usually of borderline intellectual function and are in dependent relationships with a psychotic individual.

Secondary Psychotic Disorders

The secondary psychotic disorders include those that can be attributed to a general medical condition or to the use of a recreational drug or medicine. Secondary psychotic disorders are diagnosed when psychotic symptoms occur outside the context of delirium.

CAUSES OF PSYCHOSIS

The primary psychotic disorders are idiopathic, and their cause is unknown. Several **medical conditions** that are associated with transient or permanent psychotic disorders are listed below:

- Endocrine: hyperthyroidism, hypothyroidism, Cushing's disease, hypoglycemia

- Immunologic: SLE

- Metabolic: acute intermittent porphyria; hypercalcemia; hypocalcemia; Wilson's disease; hepatic/renal encephalopathies; mitochondrial myopathy, encephalopathy, lactic acidosis, and stroke syndrome

- Deficiencies: thiamine, niacin, vitamin B_{12}

- Neurologic: seizures, Huntington's disease, Parkinson's disease, other neurodegenerative disorders, Alzheimer's disease, paraneoplastic syndromes, stroke, neoplasm, hydrocephalus

- Infectious: HIV, neurosyphilis, infectious encephalopathies or meningitides

These **substances** may also induce psychotic symptoms:

- Drugs of abuse: alcohol, sedative/hypnotics, opioids, cocaine and other psychostimulants, phencyclidine, hallucinogens, inhalants, cannabis

- Cardiac medications: digitalis (Digoxin, Lanoxin), lidocaine (DermaFlex) and procainamide (Procan SR, Procanbid, Pronestyl, Pronestyl-SR), prazosin (Minipress), captopril (Capoten)

- Pulmonary/ENT medications: steroids and steroid inhalers

- Psychiatric medications: anticholinergic medications (benztropine [Cogentin], diphenhydramine [Benadryl, Benylin], trihexyphenidyl [Artane, Artane Sequels, Trihexane, Trihexy-2, Trihexy-5]), psychostimulants

- GI medications: cimetidine (Tagamet, Tagamet HB)

- NSAIDs

- Endocrine medications: thyroid supplements and steroids

- Neurologic medications: amantadine (Symadine, Symmetrel), bromocriptine (Parlodel), levodopa (Dopar, Larodopa)

- Heavy metals and pesticides

ASSESSMENT

Initial assessment of psychosis is focused on accurate diagnosis through a careful medical history, psychiatric history, and mental status exam. The differential diagnosis includes primary and secondary psychotic disorders, mood disorders, personality disorders (especially cluster A and borderline personality disorder), delirium, and dementia.

HPI

- Inquire about the onset and time course of symptoms. Schizophrenia usually has a prodromal phase characterized by negative symptoms and odd beliefs or behaviors that may last years before onset of overt psychotic symptoms. Abrupt onset secondary to recent psychosocial stressor suggests brief reactive psychosis and comorbid personality disorder. Abrupt onset may also coincide with substance use or medicine changes and suggests a substance-induced disorder. Previous episodes with complete remission are more consistent with a mood disorder, whereas chronic deterioration since onset is more suggestive of schizophrenia.

- Inquire about previous episodes. How were they treated? How long did they last? Did they require hospitalization? Were there mood symptoms?

- Inquire about current illicit substance and alcohol use. Even if the patient has a primary psychotic disorder, treatment is ineffective if chemical dependency issues are unresolved.

- Inquire about suicidal ideation and history of suicide attempts.

- Inquire about homicidal ideation, history of violence, and the patient's perception regarding his personal safety. Scared or paranoid patients may be at a high risk for preemptive violence, especially if persecutory delusional themes involve people in their household.

PMH

- Inquire about history of medical illness associated with psychotic disorders.

MEDS

- Inquire about any recent changes in medications associated with psychotic symptoms.

- Inquire about patient compliance with antipsychotic medication.

FH

- Family history can aid in diagnosis if a psychotic patient has prominent mood symptoms.

- Family history of sociopathy, criminal behavior, etc., or of somatization disorder suggests personality disorder.

- Family history of suicide is a suicide completion risk factor.

- Family history of alcoholism suggests possible substance dependence.

SOC

- Inquire about premorbid function and best level of function.

- Inquire about chemical abuse or dependency.

- Inquire about social support structure and current stressors.

PE

- A complete physical and neurologic exam is critical.

- Exam should focus on physical findings that suggest secondary psychosis.

- Baseline weight is useful before initiating antipsychotic medications.

MSE

Note both positive and negative symptoms:

- GAB: Patients may be dirty and apathetic, with odd posturing. They may be uncooperative and negativistic. They may have evidence of tardive dyskinesia or a Parkinsonian tremor secondary to antipsychotic medications. In contrast, they may exhibit frank agitation. Eye contact may be a fixed, unblinking stare, or patients may look suddenly around the room as if responding to voices.

- SP: May be regular. Mutism is a common negative symptom. Patients may have a long latency as they edit thoughts or attend to auditory hallucinations. Disorganized speech can take the form of "word salad."

- TP: May exhibit blocking, a common negative symptom, or may exhibit a formal thought disorder with loosening of associations.

- TC: Patients may have a poverty of content or may exhibit psychotic symptoms (see the discussion of Schneiderian first-rank symptoms in Clinical Features). Well-systemized and global bizarre delusions are common. Auditory and somatic hallucinations are also common. Vivid visual hallucinations suggest secondary psy-

chosis. Auditory hallucinations that lateralize or grow louder as the patient approaches them suggest malingering. Multimodal hallucinations (e.g., "little green men that speak") are very uncommon and suggest secondary psychosis or malingering. Inquire about ideas of reference from the media (TV or newspaper) and suicidal and homicidal thoughts.

- Mood: May report incongruous mood (e.g., "I'm fine" despite being persecuted by the FBI).

- AFF: May be blunted or flat, or the patient may laugh inappropriately. Lability, irritability, and anger can occur with frightened patients.

- I/J: Patients' insight and judgment are usually poor with regard to the nature of their illness or symptoms.

- COG: Patients are usually oriented. Psychotic patients can have deficits on memory and concentration tasks due to inattention. Fluctuations in level of consciousness suggest delirium. Patients with schizophrenia may have measurable deficits in working memory and executive function.

LABS AND STUDIES

All patients should have a primary physician to assess their basic medical needs as indicated by exam and history. The following labs and studies represent a minimal assessment for new-onset psychotic symptoms and provide a baseline health screen before initiating medications:

- CBC

- Metabolic panel and electrolytes

- Thyroid function (TSH)

- Fasting glucose

- Urine drug screen

- Serum ceruloplasmin if physical or history suggests Wilson's disease

- Neuroimaging studies if neurologic exam is abnormal.

TREATMENT [4]

- Manage psychotic symptoms with antipsychotic medications.

- The atypical antipsychotics (clozapine [Clozaril], olanzapine [Zyprexa, Zyprexa Zydis], risperidone [Risperdal], quetiapine [Seroquel], and ziprasidone [Geodon]) may offer additional benefit for negative symptoms and cognitive symptoms.

- Clozapine has superior efficacy compared to other antipsychotics and is indicated for treatment of refractory psychosis but remains a

second-line treatment because of its unfavorable side effect profile and the need for careful blood monitoring.

- Depot antipsychotic preparations (haloperidol [Haldol] or fluphenazine [Permitil, Prolixin]) are indicated for noncompliant patients with poor insight.

- Electroconvulsive therapy can be effective during acute exacerbations of psychosis if there are prominent affective symptoms, or for catatonic symptoms, but chronically symptomatic patients are unlikely to respond.

- Antidepressants and mood stabilizers are used in patients with schizoaffective disorder or patients with secondary mood symptoms or aggressivity.

- Patient and family psychoeducation play a critical role in facilitating adherence to treatment recommendations and long-term treatment planning.

- Cognitive psychotherapy and supportive psychotherapies may help patients cope with psychotic symptoms that are refractory to treatment.

- Intense community casework support may reduce hospitalization by targeting resources, monitoring treatment compliance, and ensuring the environmental safety of the patient.

CLASS NOTES: DOCUMENTING PSYCHOTIC DISORDERS

ID: This is one of multiple ED visits for DB, a 27-yr-old, homeless, black male with a 10-yr psychiatric history who presents with the police after found tampering with a car door.

SO: History was obtained from the patient who is unreliable, the police, his case manager, and old records that appear somewhat complete.

CC: "I needed locomotion."

HPI: The patient has a history that appears most consistent with schizophrenia; however, his treatment course has been complicated by noncompliance with medication and follow-up, illegal substance use, and traits of antisocial personality disorder.

The patient first began having problems as a preteen with truancy, fighting, vandalism, eloping from home, and marijuana use that meet criteria for dependency. He had multiple arrests in his teenage years for possession and sales of marijuana. He was also arrested for burglary and petty theft. These symptoms occurred before the onset of psychotic symptoms at the age of 17.

The patient's first psychiatric contact was at age 17 yrs, when he developed psychotic symptoms in the context of possible phencyclidine use. The symptoms included disorganized behavior, inappropriate laughter, auditory hallucinations commenting on his behavior, and formal thought disorder. The patient was admitted to the hospital after he set his bed on fire and was treated with antipsychotic medications with partial resolu-

tion of symptoms, although he never recovered his baseline level of function. Over the years he has been admitted more than 20 times for disorganized or inappropriate behavior and has been treated with a number of antipsychotic meds (haloperidol, thioridazine, risperidone, and olanzepine), which seem to be somewhat effective in the hospital; however, the patient has rapidly discontinued such medications on discharge. His treatment is further complicated by ongoing marijuana and crack cocaine dependency. The patient has never had significant mood symptoms, although he has become assaultive at times and has been treated with mood stabilizers. He is currently maintained on haloperidol decanoate, 100 mg, which he receives at variable intervals from the ED or a community clinic. His last injection was more than 5 mos ago.

He presents now with the police after he was arrested for breaking into a car and stealing change from the dashboard. The patient denies any hallucinations, delusions, or suicidal or homicidal ideation at this time and has no previous suicide attempts. His thought process is extremely disorganized, and he makes little sense if he is allowed to answer open-ended questions. The caseworker reports that this is his baseline mental status exam.

PMH: None.

MEDS: None recently.

ALLG: NKDA.

FH: The patient's father and brother both have schizophrenia per the old chart. No documented family history of heart disease, stroke, diabetes, or HTN.

SH: The patient was born and raised in St. Louis. He dropped out of school in the tenth grade and has never held a job. He has a history of conduct disorder symptoms outlined above. He has lived in multiple residential care facilities but has eloped or been evicted from these for disruptive behaviors and fighting. He currently is homeless but has been able to meet his needs, arranging lodging in shelters in inclement weather. His legal history is outlined above. He denies recent cocaine or alcohol use but continues to smoke marijuana 2–3 times/wk. He also smokes 3 packs/day of cigarettes. He receives income via Social Security and disability. He has no guardian.

ROS: No fever, chills, night sweats, N/V, diarrhea, shortness of breath, chest pain, cough, headache, blurred vision, diploplia, sensory loss, weakness, rash, genitourinary problems, although this review of systems is not particularly reliable.

AST: General health, disability, able to meet basic needs.

PE: Temp: 98.6; heart rate: 80; BP 126/76; respirations: 16; head: atraumatic normocephalic; eyes: sclera anicteric, pupils equal, round, reactive to light and accommodation, extraocular movements intact, disks sharp; ears: tympanic membranes clear; neck: supple, full range of motion, no left axis deviation/jugular venous distention; pharynx: nonerythematous, no exudates; chest: clear to auscultation bilaterally; cardiovascular: regular rate and rhythm, normal S_1/S_2; abdomen:

benign, bowel sounds in all four quadrants; extremities: no clubbing, cyanosis, or edema; skin: clear.

NEURO: CNs II–XII intact; no tremor; strength full in all extremities; sensation to temperature and position intact; normal station, gait, and gross motor coordination; reflexes WNL.

LABS: CBC, metabolic panel, electrolytes, TSH WNL; urine toxicology positive for cannabinoids.

MSE

- GAB: Dirty male who appears older than his age, psychomotor activity shows some odd posturing, eye contact is poor

- SP: Normal volume, reduced rate, degenerates into word salad if allowed respond at length

- TP: Significant loosening of associations

- TC: He denies hallucinations, delusions, or suicidal or homicidal ideation but appears to be responding to internal stimuli at times

- Mood: "It's cool"

- AFF: Blunted

- I/J: Poor

- COG: Alert and oriented × 3; memory: 3/3 objects at 0 and 2/3 at 5 mins; concentration: can repeat months forward and backward without error; calculation: $5 - 1.27 =$ "4.50—I don't know"; fund of knowledge: able to name five cities but only current president; bizarre, loose proverb interpretation; estimated IQ: below average.

A/P: This is a 27-yr-old male with a history of schizophrenia, currently noncompliant with medication, and with ongoing substance use problems. He appears to be functioning at his stable baseline despite this and meets his basic needs of housing and nutrition. He denies any suicidal or homicidal ideation at this time and has no previous history of suicide despite chronic risk factors of psychosis, homelessness, and substance dependence.

Psychiatric Formulation

Axis I

- Schizophrenia, disorganized type

- Marijuana and cocaine dependence

Axis II: antisocial traits
Axis III: none
Axis IV: homeless—moderate
Axis V: 40

After discussing the case with the caseworker, it was decided that the patient would not benefit from inpatient admission at this time, given the chronic nature of his current problems. The patient did however agree to a shot of haloperidol decanoate, 100 mg IM, dispensed from the ED. The patient was provided transportation to a shelter, and the caseworker agreed to contact the patient the next day through the shelter outreach program to arrange follow-up. It was recommended that the caseworker attempt to obtain guardianship to help facilitate compliance in this persistently, severely ill patient. The patient was advised to avoid drugs and alcohol and understood that he may return to the ED if symptoms worsen.

ED ROUNDS: PERSISTENTLY, SEVERELY MENTALLY ILL

The example above illustrates a common problem in emergency psychiatric care—how to plan disposition for patients who are chronically, severely mentally ill, yet are able to meet their own basic needs and, other than occasionally becoming a minor public nuisance, represent no danger to themselves or others. This population is made up predominantly of patients with schizophrenia who often have comorbid substance use diagnoses. Two ethical positions come into conflict when considering the treatment of these patients—the patient's right to autonomy and the paternalistic desire of the medical establishment to provide the best possible medical care for the patient. Clearly patients have the right to make healthcare decisions for themselves even if those decisions are in conflict with physician's recommendations. But what if the patient's judgment were compromised by factors that impair his or her ability to weigh the risks and benefits of his actions? Factors that can compromise a patient's judgment may include mental illness but can also include pressures from the patient's family, cultural issues, religious issues, and economic issues. Furthermore, there are certain situations in which civil statute law may allow the physician's judgment to override that of the patient's. In these situations, it is the physician's responsibility to act with beneficence, weighing the importance of the patient's autonomy in a calculation aimed at determining a course of action that is best for the patient. The patient's right to autonomy is subordinate only to his safety and the safety of others.

In the above example several factors weighed into the decision to discharge the patient: (a) the absence of any acute deterioration in the mental status of the patient, (b) the fact that the patient has historically been able to meet his basic needs despite baseline psychotic symptoms, (c) the ineffectiveness of short-term hospitalization to thus far impact his outcome, (d) the judgment that he was at little risk of harming himself or others, (e) the willingness of the patient to accept depot medication, and (f) the ability to connect him with ongoing case management and psychiatric follow-up. The decision to further restrict the patient's autonomy by applying for guardianship was deferred to health workers who know the patient, are more familiar with the patient's longitudinal course, and can thus better weigh conflicts between the patient's wishes and needs.

Reasons for admitting psychotic patients might include (a) an acute change in mental status with an associated deterioration in self care, (b) evidence of dangerousness to self or others, (c) acute intoxication or risk of dangerous withdrawal, and (d) to assess more fully new onset illness.

REFERENCES

1. Kessler RC, et al. Lifetime and 12-month prevalence of DSM-III-R psychiatric disorders in the United States: Results from the National Comorbidity Survey. *Arch Gen Psychiatry* 1994;51:8–19.
2. Kraepelin E. *Dementia preacox and paraphrenia.* Edinburgh: Livingstone, 1919.
3. Bleuler E. *Dementia preacox, or the group of schizophrenias (1911).* New York: International Universities Press, 1950.
4. Black DW, Andreasen NC. *Schizophrenia, schizophreniform disorder, and delusional (paranoid) disorders.* In: Hales RE, Yudofsky SC, Talbott JA, eds. *The American Psychiatric Press textbook of psychiatry.* Washington, DC: American Psychiatric Press, 1999;425–477.

10 Somatoform Disorders, Factitious Disorder, and Malingering

The body has a mind of its own.

—Mason Cooley

INTRODUCTION

Patients with somatoform disorders usually present in the ED or primary care setting preoccupied by somatic concerns for which no medical etiology can be identified. In this chapter, somatoform disorders are considered along with factitious disorder and malingering, because these three classes of diagnoses are often considered together in the differential diagnosis of patients with medically unexplained somatic complaints. Keep in mind that endorsed symptoms are not necessarily restricted to ailments of the body (somatoform symptoms) but can involve psychological symptoms as well (so-called psychoform symptoms).

DIAGNOSTIC CATEGORIES OF SOMATOFORM DISORDERS

- **Somatization disorder**
- **Undifferentiated somatoform disorder**
- **Conversion disorder**
- **Pain disorder**
- **Hypochondriasis**
- **Body dysmorphic disorder**
- **Somatoform disorder NOS**

EPIDEMIOLOGY OF SOMATOFORM DISORDERS
Somatization Disorder [1]

- Somatization disorder has clear genetic contributions with high rates of concordance among twins.

- Family studies suggest sexual dimorphism, with males developing antisocial personality disorder and females developing somatization disorder (somatization disorder is approximately 10–20 times more prevalent in females).

- Lifetime prevalence is approximately 2–3% in females and perhaps 0.3% in males.

- These patients have high rates of psychiatric comorbidity, including major depression (52%), drug abuse or dependence (12%), alcohol abuse or dependence (10%), and personality disorders (particularly cluster B). Almost half (44%) have attempted suicide.

Conversion Disorder

- Conversion disorder is rare, with a prevalence of perhaps 0.01–0.3%.

- More common in patients who are poorly educated or of low socio-economic status.

- Age of onset is usually from late childhood to early adulthood. Earlier or later onset of neurologic symptoms is suggestive of nonpsychiatric etiology.

- Most recover quickly; however, 20–25% develop new or recurrent symptoms, and many eventually meet criteria for somatization disorder.

- Good prognostic indicators include acute onset, identifiable stressor, shorter interval between onset and treatment, and presentation with blindness, aphonia, or paralysis.

- Poor prognostic indicators include personality disorder or presentation with pseudoseizures or tremor.

Pain Disorder [2]

- Few data are available on the epidemiology of this newly developed diagnostic category.

- Medically unexplained pain complaints can be found in 38% of psychiatric inpatients, and pain is a frequent complaint in psychiatric clinic populations.

- The prevalence of major depression in patients with chronic pain complaints is high, although the direction of causality is unclear.

Hypochondriasis

- The population prevalence is difficult to assess but is estimated at 3–13%.

- Symptoms are transient in one-tenth of those diagnosed, chronic with fluctuation in two-thirds, and debilitating in one-fourth.

- Symptoms may fluctuate in the course of comorbid major depression.

- Comorbid mood disorders and anxiety disorders are common.

Body Dysmorphic Disorder

• Perhaps 2% of patients seeking cosmetic surgery have body dysmorphic disorder.

• Male-to-female ratio is 1:1.

• Clinical course is chronic, but symptoms may wax and wane, with the focus of concern shifting from one physical feature to another.

• People with body dysmorphic disorder suffer low rates of marriage and high rates of divorce.

CLINICAL FEATURES OF SOMATOFORM DISORDERS
Somatization Disorder

Somatization disorder presents predominantly in women with multiple, unexplained somatic and psychological symptoms, distributed across multiple organ systems, with onset before age 30, that prompt the patient to seek medical attention or that result in impairment of social or occupational function. Despite the fact that symptoms may appear dramatic, atypical, or "fake" in presentation, it is generally thought that the patient is not intentionally feigning them and perceives them to be "real." Indeed, the patient is genuinely suffering.

Undifferentiated Somatoform Disorder

Undifferentiated somatoform disorder is diagnosed if patients have one or more unexplained physical complaints that persist for >6 mos and cause occupational or social dysfunction but do not meet full criteria for somatization disorder.

Conversion Disorder

Conversion disorder is diagnosed in patients presenting with ≥1 pseudo-neurologic symptoms (paralysis, sensory deficit, impairment of balance or coordination, pseudoseizures, or convulsions) that cannot be explained by a medical condition, and which cause social or occupational dysfunction. Symptom onset typically coincides temporally with a psychological stressor. Conversion disorder is not diagnosed if the symptom is better accounted for by another diagnosis, such as when it occurs as part of somatization disorder. Although these patients are not thought to be intentionally feigning their symptoms, they often show a lack of concern regarding symptoms that would be distressing to most people, a phenomenon known as **"la belle indifference."**

Pain Disorder

Pain disorder is diagnosed when patients present with pain that is in excess of what can be explained by a general medical condition, and of which some component is thought to be due to psychological factors.

According to *DSM* criteria, it is permissible to diagnose pain disorder in the presence of a contributing medical condition if "psychological" factors have a major contribution to the onset, exacerbation, or severity of the pain. This diagnosis is problematic in that it requires the physician to make a judgment regarding whether the patient's personal perception of the pain deviates from some norm, as all pain is experienced in the brain and is thus "psychological." Nonetheless, many patients with chronic pain from identifiable medical etiologies have symptoms that clearly worsen when they are under stress, demonstrate maladaptive "illness behaviors," and suffer disability in excess of what may be expected from the "organic" lesion alone. These patients often have comorbid substance use disorders and submit to medical or surgical procedures that place them at risk for further complications.

Hypochondriasis

Hypochondriasis refers to an exaggerated fear that benign somatic symptoms are in fact the harbingers of serious illness (e.g., that a headache is evidence for a brain tumor). These preoccupations persist despite adequate medical evaluation and reassurance, and they cause significant distress and social or occupational dysfunction. Hypochondriacal fears can occur with or without insight into the absence of a rational basis for the fear.

Body Dysmorphic Disorder

Body dysmorphic disorder is characterized by a preoccupation with an imagined defect in appearance (e.g., that one's nose is too big despite multiple surgeries to reduce its size), which causes clinically significant distress. It presents most commonly to cosmetic surgeons. Body dysmorphic disorder is not diagnosed if it can be better explained by another diagnosis (i.e., an eating disorder or psychotic disorder). Body dysmorphic disorder is a controversial diagnosis; it includes a heterogeneous group of patients with other disorders such as social phobia, delusional disorder, mood disorder, obsessive-compulsive disorder, or other anxiety disorders.

Somatoform Disorder NOS

Somatoform disorder NOS includes disorders with somatoform symptoms that do not meet criteria for any of the above somatoform disorders.

ASSESSMENT OF SOMATOFORM DISORDERS

Often psychiatric consultants are asked to evaluate patients with somatic complaints that appear to be in excess of what might be expected from a medical workup. The assessment of these patients, many of whom meet criteria for one or more somatoform disorders, requires not only a thorough interview and mental status exam at the time of consultation but also access to longitudinal information regarding the patient's medical history and psychiatric history. This information is sometimes difficult to obtain because patients with somatoform disorders often have complicated medical histories and have been treated by multiple physicians, undergoing multiple surgeries and invasive diagnostic procedures that can, themselves, lead to complications responsible for somatic complaints. For somatization disorder, the Perley-Guze symptom checklist provides a valid tool for diagnosis. A clue that suggests that the patient may have a somatoform disorder is the accumulation of several (singly, none is indicative of a somatoform disorder) "three-letter diagnoses" such as **i**rritable **b**owel **s**yndrome, **c**hronic **f**atigue **s**yndrome or **f**ibro**m**yalgia **s**yndrome, **r**eflex **s**ympathetic **d**ystrophy, **t**emporo**m**andibular **j**oint syndrome, **c**arpal **t**unnel **s**yndrome, and **m**itral **v**alve **p**rolapse. Keep in mind the high rates of comorbidity when evaluating somatoform disorders and be sure to include questions that would otherwise be used to screen for mood disorders, anxiety disorders, or psychotic disorders because these patients have psychoform as well as somatoform complaints. Do not forget to assess suicide risk, as this is a critical component of every psychiatric evaluation.

STYLE POINTERS: ENGAGING PATIENTS WITH SOMATOFORM DISORDER

One of the most difficult steps in treating patients with somatoform disorders is engaging them in a therapeutic relationship. Because patients perceive their suffering as originating from a "medical" illness, they may be very resistant to the idea of psychiatric intervention. They may view a psychiatric referral as an invalidation of their symptoms or as an indication that their physicians have given up. The following example illustrates an approach to dealing with this population of difficult patients.

MH is a 48-yr-old white woman with a long, complicated medical history who was admitted to the hospital for intractable nausea and abdominal pain. Multiple workups have revealed no significant physiologic lesion to explain her symptoms; however, she refuses to leave the hospital until "someone figures this out." Psychiatry was consulted when the patient refused to leave the hospital. The consulting psychiatrist enters the room to find the patient on the phone with her lawyer.

MH: Wait a minute. There's another doctor here.

KSG: Hi. I'm Dr. Garcia. Dr. Whosenheimer called me to see if I could help with your stomach pain. Should I come back at a more convenient time?

MH: (Into the phone) I'll call you back (hangs up). What kind of doctor are you?

KSG: I'm a psychiatrist.

MH: No way. I'm not talking to you. I'm not crazy, I'm sick.

KSG: Hey, I'm on your side. I'm not convinced that you have a psychiatric illness. In addition to being a psychiatrist, I'm also a physician.

Perhaps I can give Dr. Whosenheimer some ideas that he hasn't thought about. It sounds like you've really been suffering. When did you first start having this stomach pain?

Note: Address the patient's somatic complaints first. Get a detailed medical history of the presenting symptom.

KSG: It must be pretty frustrating that your doctors can't figure out what's causing this suffering.

MH: I haven't been able to work in almost a year and a half.

KSG: Has anything like this ever happened before? Where you have symptoms and the doctors can't figure out what is wrong?

MH: Well when I was a teenager, I was having woman problems but then they said I had endometriosis and did a hysterectomy.

KSG: Did that help?

MH: Well the first one didn't, but after they got my ovaries it got better.

Note: Continue to get medical history asking about all organ systems. Get information on the degree of disability resulting from symptoms, how they were diagnosed, and how they were treated. Remember, for the purpose of diagnosis, the symptoms have to cause impairment of function or result in treatment-seeking behavior.

KSG: Did you ever have other female problems? Heavy periods? Pain during sex? Nausea throughout pregnancy? Have you ever suffered from a lot of headaches? Was it so bad that you couldn't work or go to school? Did you see a doctor? How long did it take them to figure out what was wrong? Have you ever suffered from paralysis where you couldn't move an arm or a leg? Sudden blindness? Deafness? Were you ever unable to talk? Dizzy spells? Trouble walking? What about problems with chest pain? Shortness of breath? Palpitations? Do you have an achy body? Where do you usually have pain? Would you say you have a sensitive body? Are you allergic to a lot of medicines or foods? *Transition to questions about psychiatric symptoms.*

KSG: It sounds like you've had medical problems most of your life. That must be pretty stressful for you. Have you ever suffered from depression?

Evaluate psychiatric symptoms, including mood symptoms, anxiety symptoms, psychotic symptoms, and suicide history. Consider closing with the following statement:

KSG: It is my belief that you are suffering from stomach pain. It is my understanding that your doctors have run a number of tests, and the good news is that the results reassure them that the pain you have is not being caused by any dangerous illness—any illness that is life threatening. The bad news is that they may never be able to find a treatable cause for this pain.

It is not uncommon for doctors to be "stumped" like this. There is a group of people who tend to have a lot of symptoms involving different parts of their body, and even though it may be difficult to diagnose or treat these symptoms, they tend to come and go on their own. Experience with treating these people demonstrates that even though the symptoms are uncomfortable, they are not life threatening, and they tend to improve with time. Given the number and types of symptoms you've had throughout your life, it is my impression that you fall into this category of people.

So what can be done? We know these symptoms can come and go without any medical intervention. We also know that people with these symptoms can have problems with depression and anxiety as well. The goal of treatment by a psychiatrist would be to help you cope with the stress of having so many symptoms and to treat the depression or anxiety. Sometimes medications such as antidepressants are used. You can also learn techniques to help you live with your discomfort. At the same time, Dr. Whosenheimer will be following you very closely with regular visits so that he can monitor your symptoms for ones that he can treat successfully. You say that you were feeling better last week. Wouldn't you like to feel that way more often? If you're interested, I have an appointment available next week.

TREATMENT OF SOMATOFORM DISORDERS [3]

The main focus of treatment of somatoform disorders is the same regardless of the specific diagnosis:

- To redirect the patient from his or her many somatoform complaints toward addressing psychosocial issues complicating his or her life.

- To orchestrate the treatment process minimizing opportunities for iatrogenic injury to the patient by reducing polypharmacy and avoiding unwarranted invasive surgical or diagnostic procedures that can result in needless medical complications or new problems.

- To treat comorbid psychiatric conditions. Achieving a complete or permanent remission of symptoms is not a reasonable goal.

The treatment requires the concerted efforts of an interdisciplinary team including the psychiatrist, psychotherapist, primary care physician, and occasionally other consultants, e.g., a pain management team. Treating somatoform disorders is costly and time intensive and involves regularly scheduled appointments with the primary care physician, who conducts a physical exam. Regularly scheduled appointments help reduce excessive ED visits and the associated risk of iatrogenic injury. The primary care physician should validate and acknowledge the patient's suffering and reassure the patient that although the symptoms are uncomfortable to the patient, they are unlikely to be life threatening. The primary care physician should also act as a gatekeeper for specialist referrals to help control "doctor shopping." Finally, he or she should remain vigilant for the possibility of treatable medical illness because these patients can get ill. Psychotherapeutic interventions, including insight oriented and cognitive behavioral approaches, should focus on improvement of occupational and social function, not on the elimination of somatoform complaints per se.

CLINICAL FEATURES OF FACTITIOUS DISORDER [4]

Factitious disorder is characterized by the conscious feigning of physiological or psychiatric symptoms for the purpose of assuming the sick role. It differs from somatoform disorders in that symptoms are purposefully produced as opposed to being manifestations of some unconscious process. Factitious disorder is often difficult to distinguish from malingering, as it differs only in terms of the motivation behind the feigning of symptoms, with malingering occurring for the purpose of some secondary gain.

Factitious disorder by proxy involves the production of symptoms in another person, usually a child, who is under the care of the affected individual.

Munchausen syndrome is an extreme form of factitious disorder involving feigning of symptoms, peregrination, and the telling of "tall tales" or fantastic lies. Common clinical features include

- Pathological lying

- History of multiple hospitalizations

- History of multiple surgeries or multiple surgical scars

- Willingness to endure painful or uncomfortable surgical or diagnostic procedures

- Peregrination, or the wandering from one medical setting to another

- High level of medical knowledge or use of sophisticated medical terminology

EPIDEMIOLOGY OF FACTITIOUS DISORDER

- Very rare: <1% of all psychiatry consults from medical or surgical inpatient services

- Usually females, often in the health care professions

- Occasionally males with a history of antisocial personality disorder

- High rates of comorbidity with personality disorders (particularly borderline and antisocial), substance use disorders, malingering, mood disorders, and suicidality

ASSESSMENT OF FACTITIOUS DISORDER

Diagnosis requires a high degree of suspicion. Diagnosis is further complicated by the fact that the elements that differentiate factitious disorder from somatoform disorders or malingering (awareness of behavior and motivation, respectively) are difficult to determine. Furthermore, challenges regarding the possibility that the patient may be fabricating symptoms usually precipitate the patient's withdrawal from the treatment setting, making further exploration of motivation impossible. The following features provide diagnostic clues that the patient may be feigning symptoms; these apply to factitious disorder and malingering. Keep in mind that one can detect inconsistencies or atypical features in the patient's history or presentation, but these do not necessarily lead to the conclusion that the patient is "faking." In addition, patients simulating one set of symptoms may have another—e.g., patients who present with pseudoseizures commonly have genuine ictal events as well.

General

- Inconsistencies in historical information
- Gaps in historical timeline
- Vague or evasive answers
- Suggestible with regard to nature or presentation of symptoms
- Answers that are over-inclusive of unimportant detail
- Lack of collateral sources or refusal to allow contact with collateral sources
- History of antisocial personality disorder
- Use of an alias or other false identification
- The telling of unbelievable stories
- Changes in demeanor when the patient is not aware that he or she is being observed
- Clearly identifiable secondary gain (suggests malingering)
- Documented history of factitious disorder or malingering
- A confession from the patient

Neurologic Events

- Obtundation or coma: Eyes are forward facing in truly unconscious patients. Eyes that are elevated when opened by the examiner suggest voluntary closure of the eyes. CN abnormalities are difficult to fake. Rhythmic, repetitive, passive movement of a flaccid limb by the examiner may lead to voluntary movements by the feigning patient that anticipate the passive movement, suggesting awareness. The feigning patient may protect herself if flaccid limbs are held over her face and released.

- Pseudoseizures: Alternating, rhythmic movements of the limbs in a swimming motion are common with pseudoseizures. Pseudoseizures are less likely than real seizures to be stereotyped from event to event. They are less likely to involve loss of continence or injury (e.g., tongue biting, injury during falls). Lack of a postictal state or retention of awareness of surroundings during a generalized spell suggests pseudoseizure.

- Paralysis: Loss of function that does not respect anatomical distribution of innervation is suspicious. Lack of effort can be determined if contralateral unaffected muscles are not contracted during effort. Efforts at hip flexion should produce extension of the contralateral leg, for example. By asking the patient to move the unaffected, contralateral limb, this involuntary reflex can be used to detect movement in the affected limb of a patient who is feigning paralysis. Responses can often be elicited to pain in feigning patients but not always.

- Somatosensory loss: Feigning patients have to suppress responses to pain. Sensation loss that does not respect anatomy suggests feigning—e.g., sensory loss that does not cross the midline or loss of vibration sense on one side of the sternum and not the other.

- Blindness: Feigning patients may avoid objects placed in their path. Truly blind patients cannot engage in smooth pursuit of a visual stimulus. Feigning patients will have normal pupillary responses to light and perhaps accommodation.

- Ataxia, tremor, or loss of balance: These symptoms are difficult to maintain constantly. Feigning patients may have fluctuations in symptoms when not being directly observed. Again, falls having a potential for self-harm may be avoided. *Atasia-abasia* refers to "hysterical" ataxia, a clownish gait that actually requires a great deal of balance.

Pain

- Pain is a subjective experience; thus, it is difficult to determine whether a patient is feigning pain.

- Objective signs of severe, acute pain include elevations in BP and heart rate.

- Typically, chronic pain usually fluctuates in intensity, so claims of constant or unremitting pain should raise suspicion that the patient may be elaborating.

- Peritoneal pain is usually associated with rebound and feigning patients often lack the medical sophistication to imitate this.

- Migraine headaches are usually associated with nausea and photophobia, which may be appreciated on exam.

- Covert observation may reveal that the feigning patient appears more comfortable when alone.

Psychiatric Symptoms

- Thought disorder is very difficult to simulate.

- Typical auditory hallucinations of a primary psychotic origin occur both when people are present and when the patient is alone. They are typically brief (two- to four-word sentences).

- Elaborate, detailed hallucinations suggest a toxic origin.

- Hallucinations involving more than one sensory modality in concert ("little green men that speak") are rare in primary psychotic disorders.

- Hallucinations that get louder as the patient moves toward them are atypical.

- Delusions, because they are a fixed belief, are rarely the cause of self-referral to the ED, as patients with genuine delusions usually lack the insight to seek treatment.

- Common inconsistencies in patients malingering depressive symptoms include paradoxic hunger and a conspicuous lack of insomnia in the patient who claims he has been unable to eat or sleep secondary to depression.

Other Commonly Feigned Symptoms

- Hypoglycemia: feigned by injection with insulin. Can be discriminated from a secreting tumor by testing for plasma C-peptide levels.

- Rashes, burns, or wounds that fail to heal: Infection with atypical flora (e.g., coliform bacteria) suggests purposeful contamination. The presence of wounds on nondominant side only may reflect the patient's preferred use of one hand in injecting/applying an offending substance.

- Fever: feigned by rubbing or heating thermometer. Lack of physiologic discrepancies or paradoxic discrepancies in temp from two sites of measure (oral > rectal), or dissociation between pulse and temp may provide clues.

- Hemoptysis/hematuria: feigned by placing blood in biological samples.

- Anemia: feigned by surreptitious bloodletting, or by ingestion or self-administration of anticoagulants. Stigmata of venopuncture may provide a clue.

TREATMENT OF FACTITIOUS DISORDER

Factitious disorder is difficult to treat because confronting the patient regarding the source of his or her symptoms generally precipitates his or her withdrawal from the hospital. There are no well-delineated approaches to treating this illness, although careful documentation in the medical record may prevent iatrogenic injury. Educating family and caretakers regarding the patient's illness can be useful when the appropriate consent is granted. Treat comorbid psychiatric conditions appropriately.

CLINICAL FEATURES OF MALINGERING

Malingering is not a psychiatric diagnosis but rather a behavior that involves the purposeful feigning of medical or psychiatric illness in order to gain environmental rewards. Common goals of malingering patients include gaining admission to the hospital for food or shelter, avoiding incarceration or legal prosecution, gathering social support of the public mental health system, family or friends, or procuring disability benefits.

ASSESSMENT OF MALINGERING

Assessment of a patient for malingering requires a high degree of suspicion and involves repeated interview and observation of the patient for inconsistencies or atypical features in the patient's presentation or history (see Assessment of Factitious Disorder). It is important to stress that malingering can occur in concert with other psychiatric diagnoses, so patients should receive a complete psychiatric evaluation, including a suicide risk assessment.

STYLE POINTERS: ASSESSING MALINGERING

The following example illustrates interview techniques that might be useful in evaluating a patient suspected of malingering. The strategy involves microscopically dissecting each symptom to obtain as much detail as possible about the conditions that precipitated the presentation. Facilitating questions are used to obtain information about a possible history of antisocial personality disorder. Directed questions are used to assess how suggestible the patient is.

SM is a 36-yr-old white man who presents to the ED with a chief complaint of suicidal ideation and auditory hallucinations. The urine drug screen is positive for cocaine. The patient is observed sitting on a stretcher in the ED, eating a turkey sandwich. He is watching the baseball game on TV, apparently emotionally involved. On engagement in the interview he becomes very serious and dramatic, with downcast gaze. *(Observe the patient before engaging him in the interview and note changes or inconsistencies in behavior.)*

KSG: So what brings you to the emergency room?
SM: I'll tell you, Doc. I'm depressed, I'm suicidal, and I'm hearing voices.
KSG: How long has that been going on for?
SM: Years and years. (vague)
KSG: About how many years?
SM: Ever since I could remember. Since I was a child.
KSG: You've been depressed and heard voices since you were a child?
SM: Just about.
KSG: What brings you to the emergency room tonight? Did something change?
SM: No. I just couldn't take it anymore.
KSG: Was there a straw that broke the camel's back, so to speak?
SM: No, not really.
KSG: What were you doing today before you came to the hospital?
SM: Just wandering around, thinking.
KSG: Why weren't you at home?
SM: Well, I got into a fight with my girlfriend.

KSG: What did you fight about?

SM: Money.

KSG: Is money tight?

SM: Well, lately it is. You know she's fine when I have a job. I'm always doing stuff for her like buying groceries and paying her bills, but when I'm down on my luck she turns her back on me. Like she gets pissed off if I spend money on myself when I practically raised her kids. Anyway she sent me to McD's to get some lunch for her and her kid. I ordered and gave the counter lady a twenty. Then I went to the bathroom. When I came back she wouldn't give me my change back cause she said she'd already given it to me. She put it on the counter and someone stole it. I got so mad I left without the food. Then I didn't want to go home because I didn't have the money or the food and I started to think about how I couldn't take care of my family.

KSG: So you've been wandering around since lunchtime?

SM: Pretty much.

KSG: I thought you said you fought with your girlfriend. When did that happen?

SM: Well, I guess I did go home later on, and she wanted to know what happened, and I told her, and she didn't believe me like she never does. (Why does his girlfriend never believe him?)

KSG: It sounds like she came down on you pretty hard. What kind of a fight was it? Was it an argument, was it a screaming fight, did it get physical?

SM: It was a pretty bad one. She was screaming and throwing stuff, and I tried to get by her, and I pushed her, and she fell down. Then she called the police, and you know they always take the man away in a domestic squabble, so I just left.

KSG: It sounds like this has happened before, that the police take you away.

SM: Not since I split up with my wife, but, yeah, I spent a few nights in jail. (Suggests frequent spousal abuse.)

KSG: Is that when you started to feel depressed? After the fight?

SM: Well, I was depressed before that, but the fight made it worse.

KSG: What symptoms do you get when you're depressed?

SM: I get sad, don't want to do anything, just want to kill myself. (What about the voices? Seems like a pretty dramatic symptom to overlook.)

KSG: Have you ever tried to kill yourself?

SM: I tried to shoot myself once, but the gun jammed. On the way over here I stepped in front of a car but it swerved. I guess I can't even do that right.

KSG: How about your appetite or your sleep—do those change when you're depressed?

SM: Yeah, I can't eat anything, and I don't want to get out of bed.

KSG: But before this fight you were eating and sleeping OK. (This direct question contradicts the patient's assertion that he has been having depressive symptoms all of his life.)

SM: Oh yeah, I was doing pretty good. (This answer contradicts his previous history.)

KSG: When was the last time you had depression where there were problems with your sleep or appetite?

SM: Oh, I haven't had problems like that since I guess my dad died 5 years ago. (Perhaps he has had a major depressive episode in the past.)

KSG: So let me make sure I understand what you're saying. You've had bouts of depression in the past but were doing pretty well up until this afternoon when you got into a fight with your girlfriend and then you became depressed and suicidal. Is my understanding correct?

SM: Yes.

KSG: Now when did you start hearing the voices? (Next, a series of direct questions will be used to assess the patient's assertion that he is having psychotic symptoms.)

SM: I guess after that fight. It just comes in my head saying, "You don't have anything to live for" or "Just kill yourself." (The patient asserted previously that he heard voices his entire life.)

KSG: Is it a voice that you recognize?

SM: No.

KSG: Is it a man's voice or a woman's voice?

SM: I think it's a man's.

KSG: Do you hear it outside your head like you're hearing my voice or is it inside your head more like a thought?

SM: It's like a voice inside my head. (Auditory hallucinations are generally described as sensory events, not thoughts. This symptom may be interpreted to be more likely a form of obsessive rumination.)

KSG: Are you left handed or right handed? (The patient has no idea why I'm asking this question, but I'm asking it so it must be important.)

SM: Right handed.

KSG: When you hear the voice on the inside of your head do you hear it on the left side or the right side? (Thoughts do not lateralize in the head, but the previous question implies that they should since handedness is lateralized.)

SM: Mostly on the right side. (The patient answers the question the way he feels he is supposed to answer.)

KSG: When you hear the voice on the right side of your head do you also feel a pressure behind your right eye that shoots to the back of your head? (This would be a very atypical presentation for auditory hallucinations.)

SM: Yeah. Sort of a buzzing. (The patient is very suggestible.)

KSG: Where do you think that voice comes from?

SM: I guess it happens because I'm depressed. (Preserved insight is unusual in truly psychotic patients.)

KSG: Have you ever seen a doctor or psychiatrist about this?

SM: No, I never thought to.

Assess the patient for manic symptoms and other psychotic symptoms, dissecting affirmative answers. Assess for symptoms of antisocial personality disorder using facilitating questions. Start with symptoms of conduct disorder:

KSG: Sometimes when people suffer from depression as a child, they have problems in school or with other kids. Did you have problems growing up? Did you have a short temper? Did you get into fights with other kids? Did you win or lose? What's the worst you ever beat someone up? Did you ever use a weapon like a knife or a bat? Did you ever use a gun? Sometimes when people are depressed as kids they take their anger out in other ways, like throwing rocks at houses or windows or cars. Did you ever do that? Did you ever set anything on fire? Did you ever take your anger out on animals? Sometimes when people are depressed they avoid school or run away from home. Did you ever get in trouble for cutting school or running away from home? Did you party a lot as a teenager? Did you drink? Use drugs? Did you ever get caught? Were you ever in trouble with the police?

Continue to gather information regarding social history to identify symptoms of antisocial personality disorder. Always assess for substance use disorders and suicide risk.

TREATMENT OF MALINGERING

Malingering is not a diagnosis. The final disposition will be determined by weighing the risks and benefits of the available treatment options with respect to the patient's diagnosis. For example, the patient may be feigning psychotic symptoms to obtain food and lodging at the hospital but may be genuinely suffering from cocaine dependence and a substance-induced mood disorder. In this case, one might offer treatments that are appropriate for these diagnoses including a 30-day residential chemical dependency program, an antidepressant, or both. Regardless of your decision, clearly document your clinical reasoning in the medical record. These patients can be quite frustrating and may elicit strong counter-transference reactions from physicians. Remember to **take care of the patient.** A psychotherapeutic intervention may be required to convince the patient to accept your proposed treatment pathway over short-term secondary gain.

CLASS NOTES: DISPOSITION OF THE MALINGERING PATIENT

The following is a hypothetical assessment of the patient illustrated above:

A/P: This is a 36-yr-old man with no past psychiatric history and no collateral informants, who presents with a complaint of depressed mood, auditory hallucinations, and suicidal ideation after an argument with his girlfriend. There are several inconsistencies in his presentation that suggest he is elaborating or exaggerating his current symptoms to gain admission to the hospital. (a) The patient shows few objective signs of depression or psychosis when being observed surreptitiously—he is watching the baseball game and cheering for his sports team, he is interacting with other patients and staff appropriately, despite claims of reduced appetite, he completed 100% of his meal—but became dramatically despondent at the onset of the interview, later showing full range of affect. (b) The patient lied during the interview, initially concealing events leading up to his presentation, including his use of cocaine. (c) The patient meets formal criteria for antisocial personality disorder, admitting to symptoms of conduct disorder as a child. (d) Answers to questions regarding auditory hallucinations reveal the patient to be highly suggestible. (e) The patient refused any treatment intervention other than admission to the hospital, becoming belligerent and threatening to kill himself if he were sent to a chemical dependency treatment program.

The patient does have a history consistent with one possible major depressive episode several years ago, and he meets criteria for cocaine abuse. In general, psychosis and depression may result from cocaine intoxication or withdrawal, respectively, although there are no physiological signs of intoxication at this time. He has a number of risk factors for completed suicide including history of previous attempts, unstable social environment, and recent substance use.

Psychiatric Formulation

Axis I

- Rule out cocaine-induced psychosis and depression

- Rule out major depressive disorder

- Rule out malingering

- Cocaine abuse

Axis II: Antisocial personality disorder
Axis III: Urine drug screen cocaine positive
Axis IV: Homeless—moderate
Axis V: 40

Given these suicide risk factors and the lack of collateral information, I will admit the patient voluntarily to the observation unit and observe him for objective signs of psychosis or depression. I will hold psychotropic meds at this time, as I believe the patient is likely to improve with abstinence from cocaine. I will attempt to gather information from collateral sources. I will attempt to arrange chemical dependency treatment should the patient accept it.

The decision to admit the patient is based on the lack of collateral information regarding this particular patient. A different physician may have used different judgment and documented the diagnosis and plan to discharge the patient as follows:

Axis I

- Malingering

- Cocaine abuse

Axis II: Antisocial personality disorder
Axis III: Urine drug screen cocaine positive
Axis IV: Homeless—moderate
Axis V: 40

Despite these suicide risks, the inconsistencies in his presentation (including the fact that the patient shows no objective signs of depression or psychosis) suggest that the patient is elaborating his current symptoms and that his current suicide threat is an attempt to manipulate a hospital admission. It is my medical judgment that he is unlikely to complete suicide in the short term, although chronic suicidal ideation and impulsivity place him at increased long-term risk. Regardless, a brief admission to the hospital is unlikely to resolve chronic suicidal ideation, and there is a significant risk that it may reinforce maladaptive and dangerous coping strategies, placing the patient at higher future risk. The patient's mental health interests are best served by admission to a chemical dependency program, which the patient has refused. Therefore, I will discharge the patient with a referral to a 30-day residential drug and alcohol treatment program should he decide to exercise that option. The patient was also given a referral to a shelter, and arrangements were made for transportation.

The lessons to be learned here are that (a) different physicians may have clinically justifiable differences of opinion regarding the management of the same patient, and (b) the documentation of clinical reasoning for these patients can be time-consuming, but it is important, as it provides critical collateral information for physicians who may care for this patient under similar circumstances in the future.

REFERENCES

1. Zoccolillo M, Cloninger CR. Somatization disorder: psychologic symptoms, social disability, and diagnosis. *Compr Psychiatry* 1986;27(1):65–73.
2. King SA. Pain disorder. In: Hales RE, Yudofsky SC, Talbott JA, eds. *The American Psychiatric Press textbook of psychiatry.* Washington, DC: American Psychiatric Press, 1999;1003–1021.
3. Murphy GE. The clinical management of hysteria. *JAMA* 1982;247(18):2559–2564.
4. Leamon MH, Plewes J. Factitious disorder and malingering. In: Hales RE, Yudofsky SC, Talbott JA, eds. *The American Psychiatric Press textbook of psychiatry.* Washington, DC: American Psychiatric Press, 1999;695–709.

11 Personality Disorders

Personality is the supreme realization of the innate idiosyncracy of a living being.

—Carl Jung

INTRODUCTION

Personality refers to a combination of enduring, habitual patterns of behavior or traits that color how each person interprets and reacts to other people and life events. These traits influence our perception, affectivity, interpersonal function, and impulsivity. Some models of personality divide these traits into those that are largely inherited (temperament) and those that are acquired developmentally (character) [1]. Our temperament determines our natural tendency to seek out novel environments, avoid harmful stimuli, and respond to the praise of others, as well as our tendency to "give up" on difficult tasks. Character is described by those traits that help us adapt our temperament to the environment and include our tendency to cooperate with others; to be independently motivated; and to accept imperfections in others, the world, and ourselves.

The development of personality is complex and is influenced by genetic and environmental factors, many of which are also likely to impact the development of axis I disorders. Thus it is no surprise that some personality disorders are often comorbid features of axis I disorders. Furthermore, personality features are often coarsened by social stress, illness (both medical and psychiatric), or injury. The behavior and human interactions of a patient with an otherwise well-compensated personality may appear quite maladaptive during a depressive episode. Therefore, personality cannot be assessed from a cross-sectional presentation; it is by definition an enduring pattern of behavior. It is important that the psychiatric evaluation of such "difficult" patients pay careful attention to all of the possible comorbidities so that an effective treatment plan can be developed.

Personality disorders are characterized by an inflexible pattern of perception, interpretation, and reaction to situations, other people, and oneself. Personality disorders are coded on axis II. The *DSM-IV* attempts to outline categorical diagnoses for personality disorders, but keep in mind that personality traits fall along a continuum. Thus, narrative descriptions of personality are often more useful than specific diagnoses. Another useful exercise is to think of certain personality disorders as attenuated versions of axis I disorders. In some instances (as with schizotypal personality disorder), the diagnosis is substantiated by family studies and natural history.

DIAGNOSTIC CATEGORIES

DSM-IV divides personality disorders into three clusters:

Cluster A (odd and suspicious)

- **Paranoid personality disorder**
- **Schizoid personality disorder**
- **Schizotypal personality disorder**

Cluster B (dramatic, erratic, emotional)

- **Histrionic personality disorder**
- **Narcissistic personality disorder**
- **Antisocial personality disorder**
- **Borderline personality disorder**

Cluster C (anxious)

- **Avoidant personality disorder**
- **Dependent personality disorder**
- **Obsessive-compulsive personality disorder**
- **Personality disorder NOS**

CLINICAL FEATURES

What follows is a brief description of each personality, an example or archetype, and special considerations that should be made when treating patients with these personality disorders or traits in the hospital setting. For the complete diagnostic criteria, see the *DSM* [2].

Cluster A Personality Disorders (Odd and Suspicious)
Paranoid Personality Disorder

- Archetype: the bigot
- Analogous axis I disorder: delusional disorder

Patients are preoccupied with suspicions that they are being exploited, harmed, or deceived by others. They are distrustful, unforgiving, and grudge bearing. They tend to perceive threatening meanings in remarks that appear benign to others and react harshly with anger or counterattack. In treating patients with these personality traits, provide special care to issues of confidentiality and informed consent. Carefully explain changes in treatment plan before initiation. Discuss all results promptly with the patient along with the possible interpretations.

Schizoid Personality Disorder

- Archetype: the computer geek

- Analogous axis I disorder: schizophrenia (negative symptoms)

Patients are characterized by a lack of desire for social interaction. People with schizoid traits tend to be loners, uninterested in close relationships of any kind, and indifferent to the praise or criticism of others. They may appear cold and emotionless, with a flattened affect. These patients tend to underreport medical illness and often present after illness has progressed. When dealing with these patients, physicians should be aware that they minimize complaints.

Schizotypal Personality Disorder

- Archetype: the fortune teller
- Analogous axis I disorder: schizophrenia (positive and negative symptoms)

Patients have personality traits similar to schizoid patients but are also influenced by odd beliefs, magical thinking, ideas of reference, suspiciousness, and unusual perceptual experiences. They may dress eccentrically and exhibit odd speech or thought patterns. These patients may be inclined to seek mystical remedies and alternative medicines or to ascribe magical meanings (e.g., "bad karma") to illness.

Cluster B Personality Disorders (Dramatic, Erratic, Emotional)

Cluster B personality disorders (particularly borderline and antisocial personality disorders) comprise a significant proportion of inpatient populations and use ED services frequently. Therefore, special attention is paid to these disorders.

Narcissistic Personality Disorder

The archetype is the prince or princess. Patients have an exaggerated sense of importance and entitlement and are given to vanity and envy. Constantly comparing themselves against others, they perceive themselves as separate and special and will often feel deserving or slighted. They lack empathy and will be interpersonally exploitive, taking advantage of others. In the hospital, these patients will disparage their physicians, often demanding to see a specialist. In treating these patients, the physician must be validating of the patient's emotional needs but also set limits to avoid being perceived as weak or inferior by the patient.

Histrionic Personality Disorder

The archetype is the actor or actress. Histrionic people are comfortable only when they are the center of attention. They tend to interact in a seductive or provocative manner. They tend to be dramatic, both verbally and emotionally, using superlatives and exaggerated body language. They tend to overestimate the intimacy of relationships. They are suggestible and easily influenced by others. Of all of the personality disorders, these patients are relatively easy to treat because of their responsiveness (albeit of short duration) to attention and praise. Physicians must be careful, however, to avoid professional boundary violations because of the seductive nature of these patients.

Antisocial Personality Disorder

The archetype is the confidence artist. Patients are frequent users of ED services and usually present with substance use disorders, disturbances of mood, or impulse control issues. They are at increased risk for violence and suicide. Their diagnosis and treatment are complicated because they often exaggerate existing symptoms or even fabricate symptoms to achieve secondary gain. Antisocial personality disorder by definition is preceded by a history of conduct disorder as a child. Patients with antisocial personality disorder demonstrate impulsivity, irritability, and a disregard for social norms and the safety and feelings of others, coupled with an absence of remorse.

Clinical management of these patients is difficult because their tendency toward manipulation and deceit interferes with the ability to establish a stable therapeutic relationship. Nonetheless, these patients often require treatment of comorbid psychiatric conditions that further predispose them to dangerous behavior. This treatment is best accomplished in a structured, closed environment that provides clear boundaries and consequences and that forces the patient to take responsibility for his behaviors.

Borderline Personality Disorder [3]

The archetype is the "fatal attraction" and is characterized by instability of affect, self-image, and relationships. These patients frequently use health care resources, including ED visits and hospitalizations. Chronic feelings of emptiness and boredom are coupled with intense emotional lability. This instability applies also to the patient's self-image and perception of others, which may rapidly alternate between idealized and devalued states. The borderline personality can be best characterized as "stably unstable," with frequent and severe decompensation in the face of crises that might be perceived by others to be minor. During these decompensations, patients may engage in both self-harming and suicidal behaviors.

Patients with borderline personality disorder are the most difficult psychiatric patients to treat. The prevalence of comorbid psychiatric disorders is high, particularly mood disorders, anxiety disorders, substance use disorders, and somatization disorder. The presenting picture of these axis I disorders is contaminated by the unstable nature of the personality; thus, it is difficult to distinguish between acute decompensation due to worsening axis I illness or due to the fluctuations in behavior inherent to the personality disorder. This ambiguity, coupled with a high rate of completed suicide (approximately 10%), complicates treatment and disposition planning.

Treatment involves providing frequent contact and supportive validation of the patient's chronic suffering while encouraging the patient to take responsibility for his own behavior [4]. Evaluate suicide threats seriously, but make efforts to avoid overreaction and prolonged hospitalization because (a) the risk for suicide completion is chronic and unlikely to respond to hospital interventions and (b) hospitalizing a patient with habitual suicidal behavior in response to social stress may reinforce the suicidal behavior by moving responsibility for controlling the suicidal impulses from the patient to the physician. Brief (24-hr) hospitalizations may be necessary if the patient is severely decompensated, posing an increased acute risk. Clearly address the expectations of the patient regarding the purpose and duration of the hospitalization, and set and adhere to firm limits. The issues of chronic suicidal ideation and suicide risk assessment are addressed in Chap.12, Suicide Risk Assessment.

Cluster C Personality Disorders (Anxious)

Avoidant Personality Disorder

- Archetype: the wallflower

- Analogous axis I disorder: social phobia

Avoidant personality disorder describes people who avoid activities and involvement with other people because of the fear of criticism or ridicule. These patients feel a sense of social inadequacy that inhibits them in social situations and prevents them from trying new things or meeting new people. Avoidant patients may delay seeking treatment of medical illnesses for fear of criticism. They may also underreport symptoms. Approach these patients privately in the medical setting. The use of sincere praise and positive reinforcement may be effective in putting them at ease.

Dependent Personality Disorder

- Archetype: the clingy housewife

- Analogous axis I disorder: generalized anxiety disorder with agoraphobia

Dependent personality disorder is characterized by an excessive need to be cared for by others. As a result, these patients tend to develop relationships in which they assume a subordinate position. They are indecisive, usually looking to others to make decisions for them. They are unable to initiate or complete projects on their own. They are hesitant to disagree with others for fear of losing support. When these patients present in the medical setting, they look to physicians or family to make decisions for them. The patient's indecision may be addressed by showing the patient that regardless of what medical decisions are made, the treating physician will remain available to provide care.

Obsessive-Compulsive Personality Disorder

- Archetype: the schoolmaster/the file clerk

- Analogous axis I disorder: obsessive-compulsive disorder

Obsessive-compulsive personality disorder is characterized by behavior that reflects a preoccupation with orderliness, perfection, and control at the expense of efficiency and flexibility. Patients cannot see the forest for the trees. Their preoccupation with details and rules and their insistence on perfection often disrupts their ability to complete work in a timely fashion. They tend to be scrupulously observant to rules and inflexible about issues of morality, ethics, or values. They are misers and packrats, unwilling to spend money or discard useless or worn out objects. They are rigid and stubborn. In the medical setting, these patients' personalities are liable to coarsen further due to the inherent lack of control. These patients are made more comfortable if they are provided with information and choices to restore their sense of self-control.

STYLE POINTERS: ASSESSING PERSONALITY DISORDER

Because personality disorders are lifelong patterns of behavior, they cannot be diagnosed based on a cross-sectional observation of a patient's behavior. Certain lines of questioning can elucidate patterns of behavior that are indicative of personality disorders. Accurate information can usually be gathered with the use of facilitating and normalizing questions. Use the patient's chief complaint as a springboard. Start with mild symptoms and escalate questions toward more severe symptoms. The following line of questioning could be used to ask about **conduct disorder** symptoms, for example:

- Sometimes when people are depressed from an early age, they will have other problems with their behavior as children. Did you ever have problems with your temper? Did it ever cause you to get into fights? Did you usually win or lose your fights? What was the worst you ever beat someone up? Did you ever use a weapon like a club, knife, or gun? Sometimes depressed kids will show their depression and anger in other ways. For example, they will break things, such as throwing rocks through windows, keying cars, setting stuff on fire. Did you ever do stuff like that? Did you have problems in school? Did you ever skip school or run away from home? Were you ever arrested as a child?

Questions about **borderline behaviors** may follow this example:

- Sometimes when people get depressed they develop "depressed-people habits" and ways of viewing life and dealing with stress. For example, people will hurt themselves to relieve stress. Have you ever cut or burned yourself, not to kill yourself but to relieve stress? Have you ever hurt yourself to show others how bad you feel? Do you tend to be "all or none" with regard to relationships? Do the people you love frequently disappoint you? Do you have a temper? Do you find it difficult to control? (**Note:** The phrasing at the beginning of these vignettes facilitates the answer by normalizing the patient's experience to the experiences of other "hypothetically" depressed people. It assumes a causal etiology between "depression" and borderline or conduct disordered behavior that has not been established empirically. However, framing the illness to the patient in this way may facilitate the information gathering process and begins to establish in the patient's mind the distinction between "feeling" and "behaving.")

These sorts of questions, along with careful observation of social history with regard to relationships, work history, and legal problems, help develop a profile of the patient's personality traits. Of course, the most valuable information about personality can be derived from longitudinal experience with the patient and history from collateral sources.

TREATMENT [5]

- The treatment of personality disorders depends on being able to establish common therapeutic goals with the patient and working toward those goals. Because patients with these disorders typically lack insight, attributing their difficulties to the shortcomings of others, this can be a major task.

- Psychotherapeutic approaches show modest efficacy when maintained.

- Pharmacologic approaches involve treating comorbid conditions as they manifest and are not a substitute for ongoing psychotherapeutic intervention.

- The use of antipsychotic medications in cluster A disorders may impact odd beliefs and paranoid ideation.

- SSRIs may have benefit in cluster C disorders treating anxiety symptoms.

- Cluster B disorders are often treated symptomatically using antidepressants and mood stabilizers for mood lability and antipsychotics for stress related paranoia and aggression. Use benzodiazepines with caution because of the high incidence of substance use disorders in this population.

REFERENCES

1. Cloninger CR, Svrakic DM. Integrative psychobiological approach to psychiatric assessment and treatment. *Psychiatry* 1997;60:120–141.
2. The American Psychiatric Association. *Diagnostic and statistical manual of mental disorders,* 4th ed. Washington, DC: American Psychiatric Association, 2000.

3. Oldham JM, et al. Practice guidelines for the treatment of borderline personality disorder. *Am J Psychiatry* 2001;158[Suppl 10]:1–52.
4. Linehan MM. Dialectic behavioral therapy for borderline personality disorder: theory and method. *Bull Menninger Clinic* 1987;51(3):261–276.
5. Kapfhammer H-P, Hippius H. Pharmacotherapy in personality disorders. *J Personality Disord* 1998;12(3):277–288.

Difficult
Situations

12 Suicide Risk Assessment

There is but one truly serious philosophical problem, and that is suicide.
—*Albert Camus*

INTRODUCTION

Suicide represents one of the few psychiatric emergencies for which evaluation and treatment remains the proprietary domain of psychiatrists. Suicidal ideation is the most common psychiatric complaint presenting to the ED and is the complaint most likely to precipitate a psychiatric consult from the ED. Relative to the frequency with which suicidal ideation presents to the ED, suicide completion is a rare event and is thus difficult to predict. Evaluation of suicidal ideation starts with an assessment of the patient's risk factors for suicide completion. Next, the physician makes a clinical judgment regarding the risk of suicide completion for that individual. Finally, a judgment is made regarding which course of treatment best serves the patient's interest by minimizing that risk. Suicidal ideation can be chronic or acute.

ACUTE SUICIDAL IDEATION [1–6]

Suicidal ideation exists in patients along a continuum from passive thoughts or wishes for death at one end and intent, plan, and purposefully obtained means at the other. The goals of the suicide risk assessment are (a) to determine where the patient falls along this continuum, (b) to determine what precipitated the transitions along the continuum, and (c) to determine the burden of risk factors for completed suicide.

Medical Risk Factors

- Psychiatric illnesses
- Alcohol (especially) and other drug use
- Medical illnesses, especially terminal illnesses, those that are associated with chronic pain, and in patients with a high burden of illness
- Psychosis (especially with command hallucinations in the voice of an important figure in the patient's life)

Historical Risk Factors

- Previous attempts
- Family history of suicide
- History of impulsivity

Epidemiologic Risk Factors

- Male

- Age >40

- Single or recently divorced

- Unskilled and unemployed

- Access to lethal means

- Criminal offenders facing incarceration, especially for violent or sexual offenses perpetrated against a spouse or children

CHRONIC SUICIDAL IDEATION

Chronic suicidal ideation generally occurs in patients with personality disorders (usually borderline personality disorder) but can also occur with other chronic psychiatric illnesses including chronic major depression, schizophrenia, or anxiety disorders. Patients with chronic suicidal ideation may engage in frequent self-harming behaviors such as cutting themselves, burning themselves, or ingesting pills. These behaviors are not always intended to be lethal but rather are an attempt to modulate the individual's affect or to rally social support from friends, family, or the medical community. Regardless of the intent of these behaviors, acute suicide risk can coexist with chronic suicidal ideation, and patients with chronic suicidal ideation have a sustained risk of completing suicide [6].

Therefore, the management of chronically suicidal patients becomes a dilemma. They typically present to the ED in crisis, usually precipitated by some perceived abandonment, either after harming themselves or with strong feelings that they are likely to harm themselves in the near future. They may be ambivalent regarding their suicidal intent. They may alternate between minimizing suicidal behavior, rebuffing the physician's attempt to rescue them, and exaggerating it, with accompanying accusations that the physician is disinterested in their welfare. Thus, the physician is compelled to make disposition determinations based on information from the patient that appears to lack internal consistency.

Coupled with this variable presentation is the lack of data informing clinical decisions for this population. Neither long-term nor short-term hospitalization has been demonstrated to change the rate of suicide completion for these patients, who seem to maintain a risk of completion of about 1%/yr [6]. Intuitively, hospitalizing patients who use suicidal behaviors to manipulate their environment reinforces the behavior and absolves the patient of the responsibility of managing suicidal or self-destructive urges. Because chronic suicidal ideation is by definition chronic, admission to the hospital merely delays (or "turfs" to another practitioner) the inevitable decision to discharge a suicidal patient. Alternatively, admissions can precipitate a rapid, spontaneous remission of suicidal ideation that reemerges virtually immediately upon discharge. The "stably unstable" nature of this patient population therefore demands a treatment approach that is flexible and can be tailored to the presentation of the specific patient. As usual, the ability to carefully document one's clinical judgment with confidence is the best tool one can have in managing this contentious population.

EVALUATING SUICIDAL IDEATION

- Patients expressing suicidal ideation should remain on close observation and elopement protocols until they can be evaluated and psychiatrically cleared.

- Intoxicated patients who are suicidal should be detained until they are sober and then reevaluated.

- Perform a complete psychiatric evaluation of the patient.

- Obtain collateral information from prior charts, the patient's family, and the treating physician (can be done without the patient's consent if necessary because the patient is experiencing an emergency medical condition that requires evaluation).

- Perform an assessment of acute suicide risk as outlined above.

- Carefully document that the risk, benefits, and alternatives to the treatment plan were considered, that provisions were made to protect the patient, and that timely follow-up was arranged if the patient is discharged.

STYLE POINTERS: INTERVIEWING THE SUICIDAL PATIENT

It is a myth that discussing suicide precipitates ideation. Evaluate all patients for suicidal ideation. The use of facilitating questions helps normalize the patient's experience. Start with questions addressing the mild end of the suicide spectrum and move gradually toward questions regarding the more severe symptoms. Ask about risk factors. Finally, ask questions about what gives the patient hope or what has prevented him or her from completing suicide thus far. Listen to the patient empathetically; do not try to talk the patient out of his or her suicidal ideation. The following set of questions illustrates this progression:

- Sometimes when people are depressed they feel as though "this is how things are, and they will never get better." Have you ever felt that way? Sometimes when people are depressed they feel like they can't go on, or as though they would be better off dead. Do you ever feel that way? Have you ever thought of hurting or killing yourself? Have you ever tried before? What did you do? Why didn't you succeed? Did someone stop you? Are you feeling that way now? What did you plan to do this time? How far did you get? Did you buy a gun? Did you load it? Put it to your head? What stopped you? What do you have to live for?

ED ROUNDS: DISPOSITION OF THE SUICIDAL PATIENT

The disposition plan for the suicidal patient is ultimately determined by a clinical judgment as to whether the patient is at risk for completing suicide in the near future. Such a judgment must take into consideration the following:

- The quality of information: Lack of collateral informants warrants more conservative clinical decisions.

- Suicide risk factors: Does the patient bear a high burden of risk? Are there acute changes in the risk profile of the patient? Are active risk factors likely to resolve with hospitalization, or is the risk of a more chronic nature?

- Presence of internal controls: Does the patient have the will or ability to overcome suicidal urges? Psychotic or impulsive patients, for example, may lack internal controls secondary to poor insight or judgment. Never release intoxicated patients from the hospital.

- Presence of or need for external controls: Could the patient be released with supervision of family? Would the patient be safer on a structured open hospital unit? Does the patient require commitment in a locked psychiatric unit?

- Biopsychosocial stability: Are the patient's psychiatric and environmental risk factors likely to deteriorate, to remain stable, or to improve in the near future?

- If the patient has already attempted suicide: Was the attempt intended to be lethal? Was it planned or impulsive? Have the circumstances precipitating the attempt resolved? Does the patient endorse suicidal ideation at this time? Are there family members who can supervise compliance with follow-up?

Whatever the clinical decision, it is important for the physician to carefully document the factors that were considered. If the patient is discharged, arrange follow-up and ensure the patient's safety by recruiting external controls (such as a family caretaker) or internal controls (such as providing the patient with explicit instructions to return to the ED or call a crisis hotline should symptoms worsen).

CLASS NOTES: DOCUMENTING THE SUICIDAL PATIENT'S DISPOSITION

The following are examples of commonly encountered situations in which careful documentation is especially important. Keep in mind that every situation is different; make decisions on a case-by-case basis.

Example 1

A chronically suicidal patient with a documented psychiatric history and multiple previous suicide attempts is self-referred to the ED after she cut her wrists with a razor. She has four superficial lacerations that have been sutured with two sutures. Her acute decompensation was precipitated by a fight with her boyfriend. On initial presentation to the ED she was intoxicated but is currently sober. Despite the patient's claim that she remains suicidal, you feel her discharge is appropriate.

A/P: This is one of many ED visits for this patient with a documented history of borderline personality disorder and major depression, who presents acutely decompensated after an argument with her boyfriend. She states that ongoing depressive symptoms were well controlled until the argument this evening, but now she is suicidal and depressed. Her suicide risk factors include a psychiatric diagnosis of alcohol abuse (currently sober), previous suicide attempts, and recent separation from her boyfriend; however, these appear to be chronic risk factors in this patient. She has a pattern of self-harming behaviors and suicide attempts in response to similar altercations with her significant others. Her suicidal ideation rapidly resolves on admission to the hospital and reemerges shortly after discharge suggesting that hospitalization has been an ineffective tool in managing this behavior. Furthermore, hospitalization may have the unintended effect of reinforcing maladaptive behavior in this patient. While this patient is at increased long-term risk for suicide completion, it is my judgment that the adverse clinical impact of admitting this patient outweighs the likely benefits with regard to the management of long-term suicide risk.

The patient will therefore be discharged to her home with follow-up next week with her primary psychiatrist. I provided brief supportive therapy emphasizing the need for the patient to take responsibility for her behaviors. She agreed not to call her boyfriend tonight. The patient is aware that she may call the crisis hotline or return to the ED if symptoms worsen. The case was discussed with the treating psychiatrist.

Example 2

A patient presents 2 wks after the diagnosis of his first major depressive episode with his family, who asserts that he has been behaving strangely. They are concerned that he might be suicidal. In the ED he has attempted to elope. The patient has no previous suicide risk factors and is minimizing his family's concerns. You feel strongly that the patient should be admitted, and the patient refuses.

A/P: This is the first ED presentation for this patient recently started on treatment for major depressive disorder, who presents with his family after a holiday meal. The patient asserts that his depressive symptoms have resolved, but the family has noted continued sleep disturbance, weight loss, and crying spells. Today the patient read a letter at dinner thanking the family for their support despite his multiple failures. He purchased expensive gifts with money he was planning to use for college. The patient denies suicidal ideation at this time and is minimizing his mood symptoms, although objectively he appears depressed. He is refusing admission to the hospital and attempted to elope without evaluation.

The discrepancy between the patient's and family's report of symptoms, combined with the unusual recent behavior of the patient is concerning for an impending suicide attempt, despite his assertion that he is not suicidal. It is my clinical judgment that this presentation warrants further evaluation. I will therefore admit the patient involuntarily for further evaluation and treatment. The patient's family will be asked to fill out an affidavit documenting their observations. The patient will be placed on suicide and elopement precautions.

REFERENCES

1. Guze SB, Robins E. Suicide and primary affective disorders. *Br J Psychiatry* 1970;117:437–438.
2. Murphy GE. Clinical identification of suicidal risk. *Arch Gen Psychiatry* 1972;27:356–359.
3. Motto JA. Suicide attempts: a longitudinal view. *Arch Gen Psychiatry* 1965;13:516–520.
4. Patterson WM. Evaluation of suicidal patients: the SAD PERSONS scale. *Psychosomatics* 1983;24(4):343–349.
5. Robins E. Some clinical considerations in the prevention of suicide based on a study of 134 successful suicides. *Am J Public Health* 1959;49(7):888–899.
6. Paris J, Brown R, Nowlis D. Long-term follow-up of borderline patients in a general hospital. *Compr Psychiatry* 1997;28(6):530–535.

13 The Agitated, Assaultive, or Homicidal Patient

Murder, though it have no tongue, will speak . . .
—Hamlet, *act II scene 2*

INTRODUCTION

This topic deals with patients who present with violent behavior or with the threat of impending violence. It is a heterogeneous population composed of patients who may have no identifiable psychiatric disorder, those with primary psychiatric conditions, and those with mental status changes secondary to medical conditions or toxic agents. Likewise, the motivations precipitating violence are highly variable and can stem from real or perceived conflict or from impairments in communication. Violence can also be purposeless and unmotivated. The main short-term goal of treating the violent patient is to ensure the safety of the patient and the potential victims [1–3].

CLINICAL FEATURES OF AGITATION

Agitation refers to a state of increased arousal, motor activity, and emotional distress. Signs of agitation can forewarn impending violence and include the following:

- Pacing
- Fidgeting
- Restlessness
- Removing IV, Foley catheter, or other medical instrumentation
- Slamming doors or destruction of property
- Muscle tension
- Clenched teeth
- Loud or threatening speech
- Profanity

CAUSES OF AGITATION

- Intoxication, especially with disinhibiting agents (e.g., alcohol and the sedative hypnotics), as well as with psychostimulants and hallucinogens
- Withdrawal
- Delirium

- Dementia and mental retardation, especially in patients with unrecognized complaints or needs such as

  - Pain

  - Infection

  - Undetected decubitus ulcers

  - Need for toileting or cleaning

  - Deviation from familiar structure

- Psychosis: command hallucinations or persecutory delusions

- Mania

- Adverse side effects or paradoxical reactions to medication, particularly high-potency antipsychotics, SSRIs, anticholinergic medications, or benzodiazepines

EVALUATION AND TREATMENT [4]

- Agitated patients deserve a thorough medical and psychiatric workup directed toward ruling out potentially lethal toxic or general medical causes. Once identified, treat these conditions appropriately.

- Search agitated patients for potential weapons, and place them in a quiet, safe environment in which security is readily available if not physically present.

- Never interview an agitated patient in a secluded environment.

- Always have access to an escape route should the patient's behavior escalate.

- First offer patients pharmacologic sedatives if agitation is interfering with the evaluation.

- If the patient refuses medication and represents a danger to himself or others, he may be restrained and medication administered parenterally.

- Acute agitation can be treated with haloperidol (Haldol), 5–10 mg, and lorazepam (Ativan), 2 mg, given simultaneously via IM injection and repeated q20–30mins until adequate sedation is accomplished. This should not be a substitute for the identification and treatment of underlying causes [5].

ASSAULT, HOMICIDE, AND THE
VIOLENT PATIENT [2,3,6–8]

Assault is the act of willfully threatening violence or causing harm to another. The definition of assault is broad and includes verbal threats and physical posturing that does not actually cause harm (e.g., shaking a fist). *Homicide* refers to the act of murder.

EVALUATION OF ASSAULTIVE BEHAVIOR

For the purpose of therapeutic intervention, assaultive behavior can be divided according to the state of mind of the perpetrator into behavior that is premeditated and directed at a specific victim (by a perpetrator who has regulatory control over his behavior) vs. undirected aggression perpetrated by individuals with defects or impairments in affective regulation or sensorium. Assaultive behavior can also be further subdivided into situations in which violence has occurred and situations in which violence is imminent. Evaluation begins, as usual, with a thorough psychiatric interview to assess what psychiatric factors are contributing to the violent behavior and what risk factors predispose the patient to future acts of violence. **Risk factors** for violence include the following:

- History of violence.

- Visible agitation.

- Affective dysregulation due to

  - Intoxication

  - Mental retardation

  - Dementia

  - Delirium

  - Other "organic" brain syndromes

  - Mania

  - Personality disorder (particularly antisocial and borderline personality disorders)

- Psychosis: Violence may be precipitated by command hallucinations, may be a defensive reaction to paranoid ideation or delusions, or a result of delusions of control. Violence is more common in nonparanoid schizophrenia (e.g., disorganized, undifferentiated), however, than in paranoid schizophrenia in the hospital setting.

- Suicidal ideation or previous attempts: Suicidal patients are at higher risk for homicide.

- Violent or aggressive personality style (particularly antisocial personality disorder).

- Isolation or lack of support system.

- Situational stress.

- Violent rearing.

- Violent fantasies or ideation.

- Available means and access to victim.

- Male.

- Age 13–45.

Next, assess the **level of premeditation.** Take a retrospective history if violence has already occurred. Violent thoughts can be categorized in the following manner, according to the level of development:

- No apparent premeditation: The patient acts explosively in an undirected fashion. This most commonly occurs with individuals with impairment in affective control.

- Undirected violent fantasies: Common and not necessarily pathologic. The key features are that the targets of violence are not specifically identified, and the patient has no intent of committing the act, nor does he sense impending loss of control over his actions, e.g., "When I'm on a crowded elevator that is stopping at every floor so that people can avoid going down one flight of steps, it makes me want to pull a 'Rambo' and kill everyone in there, but I'd never do it."

- Directed violent fantasies: Common. They differ from undirected fantasies in that there is a specified target, e.g., "When my boss tells me what to do, I just want to curl my fist into a ball and punch him in the face, but I would never do it." Fantasies do not forewarn impending violence and, thus, there is no duty to warn targets of these fantasies.

- Violent ideation: More concern for impending violence. The patient conveys concern about his ability or desire to control his behavior. Also included in this category is obsessive rumination on violent themes. Violent ideation can be directed at a particular individual or it can be diffuse.

- Intent and plan: Take seriously patients who espouse violent intent. Again, violent intent can be targeted at particular individuals or it can be diffuse.

Finally, a general assessment is made regarding the need for and the extent of external controls to be placed on the patient's behavior. For a patient with dementia who is exhibiting undirected aggression in the context of a UTI, intensified assault precautions at a residential care facility for the duration of treatment of the infection may be sufficient, or the patient may require hospitalization. Detain patients who present to the ED with violent ideation both for a complete psychiatric evaluation and to provide time for the patient to "cool down," even if there is no immediately identifiable psychiatric illness. Before release, make an attempt to warn specified targets of persisting violent threats, which entails contacting those targets directly, contacting family members or people who can otherwise warn the targets, or contacting the police if those individuals cannot be reached. Confidentiality can be breached to warn potential victims. Document these contacts in the chart along with the clinical reasoning for breaching patient confidentiality.

CLASS NOTES: THE VIOLENT PATIENT

Patients with homicidal ideation occasionally present to the ED who, after thorough evaluation, are determined to have no psychiatric condition that would benefit from further hospitalization. For example, an intoxicated patient with a diagnosis of antisocial personality disorder referred by the police is admitted to the hospital based on the assertion that he plans to kill his wife. Despite detoxification, the patient continues to express homicidal ideation, but there is no evidence of any other psychiatric diagnosis. In such a situation, there is no medical justification for the continued hospitalization, as the patient's personality disorder is unlikely to resolve, but the patient remains a threat to his wife. In such a case, the responsibility of the physician to society outweighs his responsibility to the patient, and it is the duty of the physician to warn the wife of the patient's impending discharge and of his threats. The discharge of such a patient might be documented as follows:

A/P

- Axis I: Alcohol abuse

- Axis II: Antisocial personality disorder

- Axis III: None

- Axis IV: Argument with spouse—moderate

- Axis V: 50

Despite detoxification, the patient continues to have homicidal ideation toward his wife. Adequate clinical observation has failed to demonstrate evidence of any treatable axis I pathology, e.g., a mood disorder or psychotic disorder. Some attempts have been made to reduce the patient's risk for violence, including detoxification, and the patient has been offered chemical dependency treatment, which he has refused. The patient has a history of violent behavior in the past and it is my clinical opinion that his wife may be at imminent risk; therefore, she was contacted and warned of his threat and impending release.

Key features of documenting the discharge of patients evaluated for violent behavior or intent include statements that (a) the patient was evaluated and appropriate diagnoses were assigned, (b) reasonable treatment was provided where possible to reduce risk of violence, (c) the risk of violence at the time of discharge was reassessed, and (d) named victims were warned of any persistent risks of violence to an identifiable individual.

TREATMENT OF ASSAULTIVE BEHAVIOR

- Closely supervise assaultive patients for their safety and the safety of others. This may involve one-on-one nursing supervision or other enhanced precautions.

- The use of seclusion, restraint, or parenteral medication may be necessary if the patient is acutely agitated.

- Treatment should address underlying causes or risk factors—e.g., detoxification of intoxicated patients, antipsychotic medication for psychotic patients, mood stabilization for manic patients.

- Psychotherapeutic interventions in patients with personality disorders should reinforce the need for the patient to take responsibility for his or her behavior and the consequences thereof.

- Victims of violence have the right to file a complaint with the police. Patients or health workers who are assaulted while in the hospital should be made aware of this option.

- Pharmacotherapy, including the use of SSRIs, scheduled antipsychotics, mood stabilizers, long half-life benzodiazepines, and propranolol (Inderal, Inderal LA), has demonstrated efficacy in the treatment of aggressive behavior in affectively undercontrolled individuals.

REFERENCES

1. Tardiff K, Sweillam A. Assaultive behavior among chronic inpatients. *Am J Psychiatry* 1982;139:212–215.
2. Asnis GM, et al. Violence and homicidal behaviors in psychiatric disorders. *Psychiatr Clin North Am* 1997;20(2):405–425.
3. Tardiff K. Violence. In: Hales RE, Yudofsky SC, Talbott JA, eds. *The American Psychiatric Press textbook of psychiatry.* Washington, DC: American Psychiatric Press, 1999;1405–1428.
4. Tardiff K. The current state of psychiatry in the treatment of violent patients. *Arch Gen Psychiatry* 1992;49:1992.
5. Adams F. Emergency intravenous sedation of the delirious, medically ill patient. *J Clin Psychiatry* 1988;49[Suppl 12]:22–26.
6. Binder RL, McNiel DE. Application of the Tarasoff ruling and its effect on the victim and the therapeutic relationship. *Psychiatr Serv* 1996;47(11):1212–1215.
7. Felthous AR. Duty to warn or protect: current status for psychiatrists. *Psychiatr Ann* 1991;21:591–591.
8. Moffatt GK. A checklist for assessing risk of violent behavior in historically nonviolent persons. *Psychol Rep* 1994;74:683–688.

14 Seclusion, Restraint, Commitment, Capacity, and Competency

Though this be madness, yet there is method in't.
—Hamlet, *act II scene 2*

INTRODUCTION

Sometimes impairments in the judgment of patients with psychiatric illnesses place them at risk of harming themselves or others, either by their direct actions or through neglect of their basic needs. In such situations, it may become necessary to violate the civil liberties of an individual for the safety and well being of the patient or the public. These violations may involve restraint, confinement, or even forced treatment. This topic deals with these situations [1].

SECLUSION AND RESTRAINT

Seclusion refers to solitary confinement of a patient and may be voluntary or involuntary. *Restraint* refers to the use of devices that prevent ambulation. These devices can vary in the degree to which they restrict movement. Some restraints secure the patient in a sitting or reclined position but allow the patient use of his limbs, whereas others (e.g., leather wrist and ankle restraints) immobilize the limbs as well. Seclusion and restraint can be indicated in the following situations:

- To isolate an agitated patient from inciting sensory stimuli

- To prevent a suicidal or assaultive patient from injuring himself or others

- To prevent the removal or to facilitate the placement of medical instrumentation

- To protect a patient from falls

- As a component of a planned behavioral therapy

Take steps to prevent the use of involuntary seclusion or restraint because these represent a violation of the patient's right to autonomy and may jeopardize the therapeutic relationship between the patient and the treatment team. These steps are directed at preventing the escalation of violent behavior and include

- Verbal redirection

- The use of voluntary seclusion

- Offering sedating medication to agitated patients

When using involuntary seclusion or restraint, observe the following procedures:

- Involve an adequate number of trained personnel.

- At least five team members should be available, with each assigned the responsibility for controlling either a limb or the head.

- Clearly explain to the patient what is going to happen and that he or she will not be harmed.

- Use the least restrictive methods first:

  - Offer medication before administering medication by force.

  - Allow the patient to walk to the seclusion area voluntarily before escorting the patient forcibly.

  - Use seclusion before using restraint.

  - Use the least restrictive restraint necessary to achieve appropriate therapeutic goals.

- Alternatives may be presented as a "forced choice" to allow the patient as much control over the situation as possible:

  - "Would you prefer to take the medication by mouth or as a shot?"

  - "Would you prefer to return to your room or would you like to be escorted to the seclusion room?"

  - "Would you prefer to walk or should we carry you?"

- Document the date and time of the evaluation.

- Document the behavior that the patient was engaged in to precipitate action, including a mental status exam.

- Document what alternatives were attempted before the use of restrictive methods.

- Document the steps that are being taken to mitigate the need for restraints.

- Document criteria for discontinuation of restrictive measures.

- Reevaluate the patient periodically for discontinuation of restraints.

- Discontinue seclusion or restraint in a graded fashion to allow for adequate evaluation of the patient's behavior—e.g., remove restraints sequentially, allow patient to sit quietly in the unlocked seclusion room.

CLASS NOTES—DOCUMENTING SECLUSION AND RESTRAINT

When documenting the use of seclusion or restraint, organize the information in a progress note that describes **s**ubjective findings, **o**bjective findings, **a**ssessment, and **p**lan. The following example documents the use of restraint adequately in a SOAP note.

12/1/01 19:30

S: Called to see patient with a diagnosis of schizophrenia who is throwing food trays at the staff and other patients. The patient has been progressively more agitated throughout the day—pacing, making verbal threats, and slamming doors. He has received no scheduled medication since 8:00. The patient became verbally assaultive after his request for an additional dinner plate was denied. He failed to accept verbal redirection to his room and began throwing food and trays at staff and clients.

O: GAB: disheveled, psychomotor activated, aggressive; SP: loud screaming; TP: loose; TC: evidence of delusions of persecution, states food is poisoned, assaultive ideas; Mood: not assessed; AFF: labile, angry; I/J: poor.

A: Axis I: schizophrenia, paranoid type; Axis II: antisocial traits per chart; Axis III: none. The patient is agitated, probably secondary to psychotic symptoms, and represents a danger to the staff and patients.

P: The patient was placed in four-point restraints and was given haloperidol, 10 mg, and lorazepam, 2 mg IM. Olanzepine was increased to a scheduled dose of to 10 mg bid. A standing order for prn haloperidol and lorazepam was written. The patient will remain on one-on-one supervision while in restraints, which will be removed sequentially when the patient's agitation resolves and he can accept verbal redirection.

COMMITMENT

Civil commitment is used to detain, evaluate, and treat patients with psychiatric conditions who represent an imminent danger to themselves or others, or who are unable to meet their basic needs. Although commitment laws vary from state to state, there are procedural similarities. Physicians and mental health workers should familiarize themselves with the laws in their state. The commitment process is usually divided into an evaluation phase and a treatment phase.

Detention and Evaluation

- The criteria necessary to commit a patient for evaluation usually include (a) a demonstration that the patient has a mental disorder or defect that includes substance use in some states, and (b) a demonstration that the patient is dangerous to himself or others, or is unable to meet his basic needs of food, clothing, shelter, or medical care.

- Usually requires a signed statement to be filed with the court.

- May be filed by nonphysicians in some states.

- Usually allows for the detention of a patient for a specified duration that varies from state to state (usually a few days) for the purpose of diagnosis.

- During this period, patients may refuse treatment except for treatment of emergent, psychiatrically unstable behavior (e.g., suicidal behavior, agitation, or aggression).

- This commitment cannot be repeated—the patient cannot be serially detained indefinitely for evaluation. Retention of the patient for further treatment is contingent on the findings of this evaluation.

- A second phase of commitment (usually lasting weeks) is required to force treatment.

Commitment to Treat

- Patient must have been evaluated. Criteria usually require that (a) the patient has a mental illness (usually a specific diagnosis) that can include substance abuse in some states, and (b) the patient remains dangerous to himself or others, or is unable to meet his basic needs of food, clothing, shelter, or medical care.

- Usually requires an appearance in court before a judge or mental health advocate.

- The patient is usually assigned a lawyer or ombudsman.

- Commitment period allows forced treatment of the patient for a specified duration (usually lasting a few weeks).

- A specific treatment plan is required, and sometimes the court will only approve specific treatments.

- A separate ruling is always required for electroconvulsive therapy.

These types of commitments can be repeated if, at the end of the specified period, the patient remains a danger to self or others.

These commitments are for psychiatric care only—they do not empower physicians to perform open-heart surgery on a patient who lacks mental capacity. Patients with nonemergent medical conditions who lack capacity to make medical decisions may be treated with psychotropic medications until capacity is restored under some commitment laws if the medical condition is dangerous enough to warrant commitment. After capacity is restored, the patients can refuse treatment if they so desire.

CAPACITY AND COMPETENCY

Often, psychiatric consultants are called to render an opinion on whether a patient has **capacity** to make a decision regarding treatment or whether impairments in judgment prevent informed decision. These consultations may include situations in which a mentally retarded, demented, or otherwise psychiatrically ill patient refuses treatment, requests "do not resuscitate" status, or must make an informed selection among various treatment options. Capacity is evaluated for a particular time and situation by determining the following:

- Does the patient recognize the presence of an illness?

- Does he or she understand the risks, benefits, and alternative treatment options?

- Is he or she able to manipulate the information in a logical manner that allows him to arrive at a reasoned conclusion?

If the answer to any of these questions is "no," the patient does not have capacity to make an informed decision. One can take steps to restore the patient's capacity. Alternatively, one can assign a proxy (guardian) to make the decision for the patient through civil commitment procedures discussed above (if the patient is psychiatrically ill and a danger to himself or others) or through court appointment. Remember that commitment can only be used to treat psychiatric conditions until they no longer interfere with the decision-making process, not to force medical treatment.

Emergencies

When delay of treatment may endanger the life of the patient, the physician may act in what he deems to be the patient's best interest, including forcing treatment. In such situations, it is best to contact the hospital's risk management office as well as concerned family members regarding the course of treatment; however, harm should not be allowed to come to the patient for lack of a lawyer. The emergency exception should not be used to justify a prolonged course of treatment without obtaining consent from the appropriate source.

Competency is a legal term that refers to a determination by the courts as to the ability of patients to make medical decisions or manage finances in their own interest. Psychiatrists are unable to make a determination of competency, although the courts often solicit psychiatric opinion. Patients who are declared *incompetent* are assigned a guardian or conservator by the courts who then becomes responsible for making medical and/or financial decisions in the patient's interest. Incompetent patients cannot provide legal consent to medical treatment. They may *assent*, but formal informed consent must be obtained from the guardian before proceeding with medical or psychiatric treatment. The emergency exception described above applies, however.

REFERENCE

1. Yutzy SH, Dinwiddie SH. Forensic issues. In: Guze SB, ed. *Washington University adult psychiatry*. St. Louis: Mosby–Year Book, 1997;435–443.

IV

Appendices

A   Formulary

Key: generic (*Trade*): Starting dose. Usual effective dose range. [Maximum FDA approved dose; therapeutic level] SE common side effects. Unusual or dangerous side effects! (Preparations)

DEMENTIA: ALZHEIMER'S TYPE

- donepezil (*Aricept*): 5 mg PO hs. 5–10 mg hs. [10 mg qd] SE headache, nausea, diarrhea. (5-, 10-mg tab)

- galantamine (*Reminyl*): 4 mg PO bid. 8–16 mg bid. [24 mg qd] SE N/V, diarrhea. (4-, 8-, 12-mg tab)

- rivastigmine (*Exelon*): 1.5 mg PO bid. 3–6 mg bid. [6 mg bid] SE N/V, diarrhea, dizziness. (1.5-, 3-, 4.5-, 6-mg cap, 2-mg/ml oral solution)

- tacrine (*Cognex*): 10 mg PO qid. 20–40 mg qid. [160 mg qd] SE headache, nausea, diarrhea. Hepatic toxicity! (10-, 20-, 30-, 40-mg cap)

ANTIDEPRESSANTS
Tricyclics: Tertiary Amines

- Class SE: sedation, anticholinergic effects (constipation, dry mouth, blurred vision, increased appetite, nausea). Increases intraocular pressure in narrow angle glaucoma! Cardiac conduction delays! (ECG recommended before initiating)

- amitriptyline (*Elavil*, *Endep*): 25–100 mg PO hs. 100–450 mg qd. [300 mg qd; 120–250 ng/ml] SE typical class. (10-, 25-, 50-, 75-, 100-, 150-mg tab; injection 10 mg/ml 20–30 mg IM qid)

- clomipramine (*Anafranil*): 25 mg PO hs. 150–250 mg qd. [250 mg qd] SE typical class. Seizures! (25-, 50-, 75-mg cap)

- doxepin (*Sinequan*): 25 mg PO hs. 75–300 mg qd. [300 mg qd] SE typical class. (10-, 25-, 50-, 75-, 100-, 150-mg cap; oral liquid 10 mg/ml)

- imipramine (*Tofranil*): 25 mg PO hs. 50–300 mg qd. [300 mg qd; 150–300 ng/ml] SE typical class. (10-, 25-, 75-mg tab; 100-, 125-, 150-mg cap; injection 12.5 mg/ml, 50 mg IM bid max)

- trimipramine (*Surmontil*): 25 mg PO hs. 75–300 mg qd. [300 mg qd] SE typical class. (25-, 50-, 100-mg cap)

Tricyclics: Secondary Amines

- desipramine (*Norpramine*): 25 mg PO hs. 100–300 mg qd. [300 mg qd; 50–300 ng/ml] SE minimal sedation and anticholinergic. Cardiac conduction delays! (10-, 25-, 50-, 75-, 100-, 150-mg tab)

- nortriptyline (*Aventyl, Pamelor*): 25 mg PO hs. 50–150 mg qd. [150 mg qd; 50–150 ng/ml] SE minimal sedation and anticholinergic. Cardiac conduction delays! (10-, 25-, 50-, 75-mg cap; oral solution 10 mg/5 ml)

- protriptyline (*Vivactil*): 5 mg PO tid. 5–10 mg tid-qid. [60 mg qd] SE constipation, dry mouth, blurred vision. Cardiac conduction delays! (5-, 10-mg tab)

Tetracyclics

- amoxapine (*Asendin*): 25–50 mg PO bid–tid. 150–400 mg qd [600 mg] SE anticholinergic effects, extrapyramidal symptoms. Acute dystonia! Cardiac conduction delays! (25-, 50-, 100-, 150-mg tab)

- maprotiline (*Ludiomil*): 25 mg PO qd. 75–200 mg qd. [200 mg qd] SE sedation. Seizures! Cardiac conduction delays! (25-, 50-, 75-mg tab)

Monoamine Oxidase Inhibitors

- MAOIs are contraindicated in combination with most medications that increase the availability of monoamines both centrally and peripherally (e.g., most other antidepressants.) Before starting an MAOI, allow time for elimination of discontinued antidepressant medication. Patients should adhere to a low tyramine diet.

- phenelzine (*Nardil*): 15 mg PO tid. 45–90 mg qd. [90 mg qd] SE orthostasis, sedation. Hypertensive crisis! (15-mg tab)

- tranylcypromine (*Parnate*): 10 mg PO bid. 20–30 mg bid. [60 mg qd] SE orthostasis. Hypertensive crisis! (10-mg tab)

5-HT Selective Reuptake Inhibitors

- Class SE: headache, nausea, diarrhea, somnolence or insomnia, agitation or nervousness, sexual dysfunction

- citalopram (*Celexa*): 20 mg PO hs. 20–80 mg qd. [60 mg qd] SE class effects. (20-, 40-, 60-mg tab)

- fluoxetine (*Prozac, Serefem*): 20 mg PO qd. 10–100 mg qd. [80 mg qd] SE class effects. (10-, 20-mg cap; oral liquid 20 mg/5 ml; weekly 90 mg cap = 20 mg qd)

- fluvoxamine (*Luvox*): 50 mg PO hs. 100–300 mg qd. [300 mg qd] SE class effects. (50-, 100-mg tab)

- paroxetine (*Paxil*): 20 mg PO hs. 10–60 mg qd. [60 mg qd] SE class effects, dry mouth, constipation. (10-, 20-, 30-, 40-mg tab)

- sertraline (*Zoloft*): 50 mg PO qd. 50–250 mg qd. [200 mg qd] SE class effects. (25-, 50-, 100-mg tab)

5-HT and NE Reuptake Inhibitors (Second Generation)

- venlafaxine (*Effexor, Effexor XR*): 37.5 mg PO bid (*XR*: 37.5–75 mg PO qd). 100–375 mg qd. [375 mg qd, *XR*: 225 mg qd] SE headache, somnolence, dizziness, nervousness, nausea, dry mouth, constipation. Hypertension! (25-, 37.5-, 50-, 75-, 100-mg tab; *XR*: 37.5-, 75-, 150-mg cap)

NE and DA Reuptake Inhibitors

- buproprion (*Wellbutrin, Wellbutrin SR*): 100 mg PO bid; *SR* 150 mg qd. 150–450 mg qd. [450 mg qd; *SR*: 400 mg qd] SE agitation, insomnia, akathisia, anxiety, headache, weight loss, psychosis. Seizures! Contraindicated in eating disorders or with seizure disorders. (75-, 100-mg tab; *SR*: 100-,150-mg tab)

5-HT Reuptake, 5-HT$_2$ Antagonists

- nefazodone (*Serzone*): 100 mg PO bid. 300–600 mg qd. [600 mg qd] SE drowsiness, headache, insomnia, agitation, dizziness, confusion. (50-, 100-, 150-, 200-, 250-mg tab)

- trazodone (*Desyrel*): 50–150 mg PO qd. 400–600 mg qd. [600 mg qd] SE drowsiness, dizziness, headache, confusion. Priapism! (50-, 100-, 150-, 300-mg tab)

NE and 5-HT Release Promoters

- mirtazapine (*Remeron, Remeron Soltab*): 15-30 mg PO hs. 22.5–60 mg qd. [45 mg qd] SE sedation, weight gain, increased appetite. Agranulocytosis! (15-, 30-, 45-mg tab and dissolving tab)

ANTIPSYCHOTICS
High-Potency D$_2$ Antagonists

- Class SE: Because of high D$_2$ affinity and low anticholinergic effect, the high-potency neuroleptics are more likely to cause extrapyramidal symptoms (EPS: Parkinsonism, dystonia, akathisia). Sedation, orthostatic hypotension, hyperprolactinemia, amenorrhea. Tardive dyskinesia! Neuroleptic malignant syndrome!{dose equivalents in mg}

- fluphenazine (*Prolixin, Prolixin decanoate*): 2.5–5 mg PO/IM bid. 10–40 mg qd. [40 mg qd] SE class effects {2}. Decanoate: 12.5 mg IM q3wks = 10 mg qd oral. [25 mg q3wks]. (1-, 2.5-, 5-, 10-mg tab; oral elixir: 2.5 mg/5 ml; IM: 2.5 mg/ml; Decanoate: 25 mg/ml)

- haloperidol (*Haldol, Haldol decanoate*): 1–5 mg PO/IM bid. 6–20 mg qd. [100 mg qd] SE class effects {2}. Decanoate: 100 mg IM q4wks = 10 mg qd oral [100 mg/bolus—larger doses must be given in divided injections]. (0.5-, 1-, 2-, 5-, 10-, 20-mg tab; oral concentrate; 2 mg/ml; IM: 5 mg/ml; Decanoate: 50,100 mg/ml)

- perphenazine (*Trilafon*): 4 mg PO bid–tid. 4–16 mg PO bid–qid. [64 mg qd]. 5–10 mg IM q6hrs. [30 mg qd] SE class effects. {8} (2-, 4-, 8-, 16-mg tab; oral concentrate: 16 mg/5 ml; IM: 5 mg/ml)

- pimozide (*Orap*): 1–2 mg PO qd. 2–10 mg qd. [10 mg qd]. SE class effects. QT prolongation! {1} (1-, 2-mg tab)

- thiothixene (*Navane*): 2 mg PO tid. 4 mg IM bid–tid. 20–30 mg qd. [30 mg qd] SE class effects. {5} (1-, 2-, 5-, 20-mg cap; oral concentrate: 5 mg/ml; IM: 5 mg/ml)

- trifluperazine (*Stelazine*): 2–5 mg PO bid. 15–20 mg qd. [40 mg qd]. 1–2 mg IM q4–6hrs. [10 mg qd] SE class effects. {5} (1-, 2-, 5-, 10-mg tab; oral concentrate: 10 mg/ml; IM: 2 mg/ml)

Mid-Potency D_2 Antagonists

- loxapine (*Loxitane*): 10 mg PO bid. 60–100 mg qd. 12.5–50 mg IM q4–12h. [250 mg qd]. SE similar to high potency with less frequent extrapyramidal symptoms. Mild anticholinergic effects. {10} (5-, 10-, 25-, 50-mg cap; oral concentrate: 25 mg/ml; IM: 50 mg/ml)

- molindone (*Moban*): 25 mg PO tid. 50–100 mg qd. [225 mg qd] SE similar to high potency with less frequent extrapyramidal symptoms. Mild anticholinergic effects. {10} (5-, 10-, 25-, 50-, 100-mg tab; oral concentrate: 20 mg/ml)

Low-Potency D_2 Antagonists

- Class SE: Because of the high anticholinergic effect of these drugs, they are less likely to cause extrapyramidal symptoms than the high potency antipsychotics, although EPS remain a risk. Anticholinergic side effects are significant (constipation, dry mouth, blurred vision, increased appetite, nausea). Sedation, orthostatic hypotension, hyperprolactinemia, amenorrhea. Tardive dyskinesia! Neuroleptic malignant syndrome! Photosensitivity! Pigmentary retinopathy at high doses!

- chlorpromazine (*Thorazine*): 10–50 mg PO bid–tid. 300–800 mg qd. [2,000 mg qd] IM/IV preparations are to be avoided because of increased cardiac risk. SE class effects. {100} (20-, 25-, 50-, 100-, 200-mg tab; cap: 30, 75, 150 mg; supp: 25, 100 mg; syrup: 10 mg/5 ml; oral concentrate: 30,100 mg/ml)

- mesoridazine (*Serentil*): 10–50 mg PO bid–tid. 75–400 mg qd. [400 mg qd] SE class effects. {50} (10-, 25-, 50-, 100-mg tab; oral concentrate: 25 mg/ml)

- thioridazine (*Mellaril*): 50–100 mg PO bid–tid. 200–800 mg qd. [800 mg qd] SE class effects. Pigmentary retinopathy at 800 mg qd! QTc prolongation! {95} (10-, 15-, 25-, 50-, 100-, 150-, 200-mg tab; suspension: 25,100 mg/ml; oral concentrate: 30,100 mg/ml)

Atypical Antipsychotics

- Class SE: The atypical antipsychotics differ from conventional antipsychotics in that the have a lower incidence of extrapyramidal symptoms and possible tardive dyskinesia. This is due to the fact that these drugs either have lower affinity for D_2 receptors (clozapine and quetiapine) and/or high affinity for 5-HT_{2A} receptors. With the exception of clozapine and quetiapine, these drugs may cause extrapyramidal symptoms and neuroleptic malignant syndrome, although at a lower rate than conventional antipsychotics.

- clozapine (*Clozaril*): 25 mg PO bid. 450–900 mg qd. [900 mg qd] SE anticholinergic effects, orthostatic hypotension, sedation, weight gain, hyperglycemia. Seizures! Agranulocytosis! (25-, 100-mg tab)

- olanzapine (*Zyprexa*, *Zydis*): 5–10 mg PO qhs. 10–60 mg qd. [20 mg qd] SE class effects, mild anticholinergic effects, sedation, weight gain, hyperglycemia. (2.5-, 5-, 7.5-, 10-, 15-, 20-mg tab; *Zydis* dissolvable tab: 5, 10 mg)

- quetiapine (*Seroquel*): 50 mg PO bid. 400–800 mg qd. [800 mg qd] SE orthostatic hypotension, sedation. Cataracts! (25-, 100-, 200-mg tab)

- risperidone (*Risperdal*): 2 mg PO qhs. 4–8mg qd. [16 mg qd] SE class effects, sedation, extrapyramidal symptoms, orthostatic hypotension at higher doses. (0.25-, 0.5-, 1-, 2-, 3-, 4-mg tab; oral concentrate:1 mg/ml)

- ziprasidone (*Geodon*): 20 mg PO bid. 120–200 mg qd. [160 mg qd] SE class effects. QTc changes! (20-, 40-, 60-, 80-mg cap)

MOOD-STABILIZING AGENTS

- carbamazepine (*Tegretol, Tegretol XR*): 200 mg PO qd–bid. 600–1,800 mg qd. [2,400 mg qd; 4–12 mg/ml] SE sedation, dizziness, fatigue, confusion, ataxia, nausea, nystagmus. Aplastic anemia! (200-mg tab; *XR*: 100-, 200-, 400-mg tab; oral suspension: 100 mg/5 ml; Chewable: 100 mg)

- lithium salts (*Eskalith, Lithane, Lithobid, Lithonate*): 300 mg PO bid. 600–1,800 mg qd. [0.6–1.2 mEq/L] SE polydipsia, nausea, diarrhea, abnormal taste, tremor, weight gain, rash. Hypothyroidism! Leukocytosis! Diabetes insipidus! Renal toxicity! (150-, 300-, 600-mg tab; slow-release tabs: 300, 450 mg; syrup: 300 mg/5 ml)

- olanzepine (*Zyprexa*, *Zydis*): 5–10 mg PO qhs. 10–60 mg qd. [20 mg qd] SE class effects, mild anticholinergic effects, sedation, weight gain, hyperglycemia. (2.5-, 5-, 7.5-, 10-, 15-, 20-mg tab; *Zydis* dissolvable tab: 5-, 10-mg)

- valproic acid (*Depakene*, *Depakote*, *Depacon*): 250–500 mg PO bid. 500–3,000 mg qd. [60 mg/kg/day; 50–125 mg/ml] SE weight gain, N/V, diarrhea, change in menses. Hepatic toxicity! Pancreatitis! (125-, 250-, 500-mg tab; *ER*: 250-, 500-mg cap; syrup: 250 mg/ 5 ml; sprinkle: 125-mg cap)

Anticonvulsants Used Off-Label for Mood Stabilization

- gabapentin (*Neurontin*): 100 mg PO tid. 300–800 mg tid. [3,600 mg qd] SE somnolence, dizziness, ataxia, fatigue. (100-, 300-, 400-mg cap; 600-, 800-mg tab)

- lamotragine (*Lamictal*): 50 mg PO qd. 150–250 mg bid. [700 mg qd; 200 mg qd with valproic acid] SE dizziness, sedation, ataxia, rash. Stevens-Johnson rash! (25-, 100-, 150-, 200-mg tab)

- oxcarbazepine (*Trileptal*): 300 mg PO bid. 600 mg bid–qid. [2,400 mg qd] SE headache, dizziness, somnolence, fatigue, nausea. Stevens-Johnson, rarely! (150-, 300-, 600-mg tab)

- topiramate (*Topamax*): 50 mg PO qd. 200–800 mg bid. [1,600 mg qd] SE fatigue, dizziness, somnolence, psychomotor slowing, memory impairment, aphasia. (25-, 100-, 200-mg tab)

ANXIOLYTICS/HYPNOTICS
Anticholinergic-Antihistaminergic

- diphenhydramine (*Benadryl*): 50–100 mg PO hs for insomnia. SE anticholinergic effects, may exacerbate delirium and dementia in the elderly (25-, 50-mg tab and cap)

- hydroxyzine (*Atarax*, *Vistaril*): 50–100 mg PO/IM q6h prn sedation or insomnia. [600 mg qd] SE anticholinergic effects, sedation. (10-, 25-, 50-, 100-mg tab; 25-, 50-, 100-mg cap; liquid: 10, 25 mg/ml)

Barbiturates

- Class SE: This class is rarely used anymore because of the narrow therapeutic index. Side effects include sedation, headache, "hangover" effect, motor impairment, ataxia, and dysarthria. Abuse potential! Withdrawal!

- butabarbital (*Butisol*): 15–30 mg PO tid–qid. 50–100 mg PO qhs for insomnia. SE class effects. (15-, 30-, 50-, 100-mg tab; liquid: 30 mg/5 ml)

- mephobarbital (*Mebaral*): 32–100 mg PO tid–qid. SE class effects. (32-, 50-, 100-mg tab)

- pentobarbital (*Nembutal*): 20–150 mg PO/IM/IV tid–qid. SE class effects. (50-, 100-mg tab; elixir: 18.2 mg/5 ml)

- secobarbital (*Seconal*): 50–100 mg PO hs. SE class effects. (50-, 100-mg cap)

Benzodiazepines: Short Half-Life

- Class SE: sedation, headache, "hangover" effect, motor impairment, ataxia, and dysarthria. Abuse potential! Withdrawal! {oral dose equivalents in mg}

- alprazolam (*Xanax*): 0.25–0.5 mg PO bid–tid. [4 mg] SE class effects. {0.5} (0.25-, 0.5-, 1-, 2-mg tab)

- midazolam (*Versed*): 5 mg IM/IV. SE class effects. (1,5 mg/ml)

- oxazepam (*Serax*): 10–30 mg PO tid–qid. SE class effects. {15} (10-, 15-, 30-mg tab)

- triazolam (*Halcion*): 0.125–0.5 mg PO hs. SE class effects. {0.25} (0.125-, 0.25-mg tab)

Benzodiazepines: Medium Half-Life

- estazolam (*ProSom*): 1–2 mg PO hs. SE class effects. {2} (1-, 2-mg tab)

- lorazepam (*Ativan*): 0.5–2 mg PO/IM/IV q4–8h. SE class effects. {1} (0.5-, 1-, 2-mg tab; IM/IV: 2 mg/ml; oral concentrate: 2 mg/ml)

- temazepam (*Restoril*): 15–30 mg PO hs. SE class effects. {30} (7.5-, 15-, 30-mg cap)

Benzodiazepines—Long Half-Life

- chlordiazepoxide (*Librium*): 25–100 mg PO q4–6h. [300 mg qd] SE class effects. {10} (5-, 10-, 25-mg tab and cap; IM/IV powder: 100 mg)

- clonazepam (*Klonopin*): 0.25–1 mg PO tid. [20mg] SE class effects. {0.25} (0.5-, 1-, 2-mg tab)

- clorazepate (*Tranxene*): 7.5–15 mg PO hs. SE class effects. {7.5} (3.75-, 7.5-, 15-, 11.25-, 22.5-mg tab)

- diazepam (*Valium*): 2–10 mg PO bid-qid. SE class effects. {5} (2-, 5-, 10-mg tab; IM/IV: 5 mg/ml; oral concentrate: 5 mg/ml)

- flurazepam (*Dalmane*): 15–30 mg PO hs. SE class effects. {30} (15-, 30-mg cap)

5-HT Agonist/Antagonist

- buspirone (*Buspar*): 5–7.5 mg PO bid–tid. 20–30 mg qd. [60 mg qd] SE dizziness, light-headedness, headache, restlessness, nausea. (5-, 10-, 15-mg tab)

Other Hypnotics

- zaleplon (*Sonata*): 5–10 mg PO hs. May repeat. SE (infrequent) amnesia, anxiety, depersonalization, dizziness, hallucinations, somnolence, impaired coordination. (5-, 10-mg cap)

- zolpidem (*Ambien*): 5–10 mg PO hs. SE headache, drowsiness, dizziness, nausea, diarrhea. (5-, 10-mg tab)

CHEMICAL DEPENDENCY

- buproprion (*Zyban*): 150–mg PO qd. 150 mg bid × 12 wks. SE agitation, insomnia, akathisia, anxiety, headache, weight loss, psychosis. Seizures! Contraindicated in eating disorders or with seizure disorders. (150-mg tab)

- clonidine (*Catapres, Catapres TTS*): For opioid withdrawal: 0.1 mg PO tid. 0.3 mg tid/qid then taper over 4–5 days. SE hypotension, drowsiness, dizziness, confusion. (0.1-, 0.2-, 0.3-mg tab; transdermal patch: 0.1, 0.2, 0.3 mg × 7 days)

- disulfiram (*Antabuse*): 125–500mg PO qd. Must avoid ingesting all products containing alcohol (cough syrup, mouthwash, etc.). SE Multiple drug interactions! Hepatitis! Neuropathy and neuritis! (250-, 500-mg tab)

- methadone (*Dolophine*): Opiate withdrawal: 5–10 mg PO q4hr prn withdrawal symptoms. Taper over 4–7 days. Maintenance: 80–120 mg qd. SE constipation, nausea, hypotension, bradycardia, fatigue, drowsiness, dizziness. (5-, 10-, 40-mg tab; solution: 5-, 10-mg/ml; oral concentrate: 10 mg/ml)

- naltrexone (*ReVia, Depade*): Opiate/alcohol abstinence: 25–50 mg PO qd. SE diarrhea, nausea, headache, myalgia. Hepatotoxicity! (50-mg tab)

- nicotine gum (*Nicorette*): 1 piece q1–8hrs tapered over 12 wks. [96 mg qd] (2-, 4-mg each)

- nicotine nasal spray (*Nicotine NS*): 2–4 spray qhr prn [40 mg qd] (0.5 mg/spray)

- nicotine inhalation system (*Nicotrol Inhaler*): 6–16 cartridges qd, tapered over 12 wks. (10 mg/cartridge)

- nicotine patch (*Habitrol, Nicotrol, Nicoderm, ProStep*): 1 patch qd tapered over 6 wks. (7-, 11-, 14-, 15-, 21-, 22-mg patches)

SYMPATHOMIMETICS

- Class SE: nervousness, tics, anorexia, insomnia. Psychosis! Mania! Abuse potential!

- *Adderall* (dextroamphetamine and racemic amphetamine): start 2.5–5 mg qd/bid. 40–60 mg qd. SE class effects. (5-, 10-, 20-, 30-mg cap)

- dextroamphetamine (*Dexedrine*): start 2.5–5 mg qam/bid. 30 mg qd. SE class effects. (5-, 10-mg tabs; 5-, 10-, 15-mg qd cap)

- methylphenidate (*Ritalin, Ritalin SR, Metadate CD*): 5–10 mg bid–tid or (long-acting) 20 mg qam. SE class effects. (5-, 10-, 20-mg cap)

- modafinil (*Provigil*): 100–200 mg qam. SE class effects. (100-, 200-mg cap)

- pemoline (*Cylert*): 37.5 mg qam. 56.25–75 mg qd. [112.5 mg qd]. SE class effects. Hepatotoxic! (18.75-, 37.5-, 75-mg tab; 37.5-mg chewable)

Adverse Drug Events and Side Effects

ANTIPSYCHOTICS

Most of the acute side effects in response to administration of antipsychotics are related to dopaminergic blockade in the striatum. Thus, the high-potency agents are more frequently responsible than the newer antipsychotics; however, these are class side effects that apply to all antipsychotics with the possible exceptions of clozapine (Clozaril) and quetiapine (Seroquel).

Akathisia

The subjective feeling of restlessness or inability to remain still. This side effect can be experienced both physically and psychologically. Treatment: Lower dose or switch agent or propranolol (Inderal, Inderal LA), 5–30 mg PO tid, or lorazepam (Ativan), 1–2 mg PO tid. Benztropine (Cogentin) is usually insufficient.

Dystonia

Sustained, painful contractions of a muscle or group of muscles. May involve the neck, trunk, eyes (occulogyric crisis), tongue, extremities, or larynx. Laryngeal dystonias can be fatal. Treatment: benztropine, 2 mg IV/IM, or diphenhydramine (Benadryl, Benylin), 50 mg IV/IM; may repeat in 10–20 mins if symptoms do not resolve. May use adjunctive lorazepam (Ativan), 1–2 mg IV/IM, as well. To prevent future dystonia, switch agent, lower or split dosing, or add scheduled benztropine, 1–2 mg PO, or diphenhydramine, 25–50 mg PO with dosing of antipsychotic.

Pseudoparkinsonism

Parkinsonism induced by D_2 blockade in the striatum. Symptoms include bradykinesia, hypokinesia, rigidity, and tremor. Treatment: Switch agent, lower dose, or add scheduled benztropine, 1–2 mg PO bid–tid, or diphenhydramine, 25–50 mg PO bid–tid.

Neuroleptic Malignant Syndrome

Neuroleptic malignant syndrome (NMS) is a response to D_2 blockade that is often dose-dependent but can also be idiopathic. Occurring in about 0.2% of patients on neuroleptics, NMS can be fatal. Symptoms develop over hours to days and include high fever, autonomic instability, mental status changes, leaden rigidity, elevated creatine kinase, elevated WBC count, and myoglobinuria. Risk factors include dehydration, higher antipsychotic doses, concomitant lithium use, and bipolar illness. Treatment: Discontinue neuroleptic. Supportive treatment in an intensive care setting includes continuous monitoring of vitals, aggressive hydration, and antipyretics. Pharmacologic management includes lorazepam, 1–2 mg IV bid–tid; dantrolene sodium (Dantrium), 0.8–1 mg/kg IV q6h; and bromocriptine (Parlodel), 2.5–5 mg tid. NMS may require several weeks of treatment, especially if depot neuroleptics were involved. NMS may respond to electroconvulsive therapy. After resolution of symptoms, antipsychotic selection becomes an issue. Clearly, switching to an atypical is the preferred course of treatment, with clozapine (Clozaril) being the first choice because of the low incidence of NMS with this agent; however, in the risk–benefit analysis, compliance issues may ultimately favor other agents.

Tardive Dyskinesia

Choreoform movement disorder manifesting as lip smacking, tongue protrusion, or choreoathetotic movements of the fingers, toes, limbs, and trunk that develops with chronic neuroleptic exposure or on withdrawal of a neuroleptic agent. Risk factors include advanced age, female sex, and possibly mood disorder. It appears more commonly with use of the high-potency D_2 antagonists. Treatment: There are no effective treatments. Switch the patient to an atypical agent due to lower risk of progression.

ANTIDEPRESSANTS
Serotonin Syndrome

Occurs most commonly in the context of SSRI use and is characterized by headache, nausea, diarrhea, fever, tremor, spreading myoclonus, hyperreflexia, dizziness, shivering, nervousness, and, in extreme incidents, mental status changes. Can be differentiated from NMS by the absence of rigidity or elevated creatine kinase. May occur in a dose-dependent fashion, with combinations of serotonergic agents, or idiopathically. Treatment: Discontinue offending agent. Benzodiazepines can be used to treat myoclonus. Cyproheptadine (Periactin), a serotonin antagonist, may be useful in treating symptoms, as may be propranolol (Inderal, Inderal LA).

SSRI Discontinuation Syndromes

Symptoms may include dizziness, vertigo, paresthesias, flulike symptoms, nausea, diarrhea, insomnia, and diaphoresis. These are usually benign and self-limited. Treatment: Gradually taper short half-life SSRIs (particularly paroxetine [Paxil]) when discontinuing medication.

Sexual Dysfunction

Manifests as delayed orgasm, anorgasmia, or frank impotence. Treatment: Drug holidays with the shorter half-life agents (citalopram [Celexa], paroxetine, fluvoxamine [Luvox], or sertraline [Zoloft]) may be sufficient or switch agents (nefazodone [Serzone], bupropion [Wellbutrin, Wellbutrin SR, Zyban SR], or mirtazapine [Remeron, Remeron SolTab] appear to have lower incidence of sexual dysfunction) or augment with bupropion (Wellbutrin, Wellbutrin SR, Zyban SR), 100–150 mg bid.

Hypertensive Crisis (MAOIs)

Occurs in the context of a hyperadrenergic state caused by ingestion of sympathomimetic substances (tyramine or phenylethylamine) in diet or drugs along with a MAOI. Symptoms include headache, hypertension, diaphoresis, restlessness, and cardiac arrhythmias. Treatment: Hold the MAOI. Give phentolamine (Regitine), 5 mg IV repeated prn. Do not use beta-noradrenergic antagonists, as doing so can exacerbate crisis.

LITHIUM (CIBALITH-S, ESKALITH, ESKALITH CR, LITHANE, LITHOBID, LITHONATE, LITHOTABS)
Toxicity

Symptoms include tremor, N/V, diarrhea, metallic taste in mouth, ataxia, polyuria, mental status changes, and arrhythmia. Dehydration is a predisposing factor. Treatment: Hold lithium salts, rehydrate; plasmapheresis may be necessary in extreme cases.

Tremor

Fine resting tremor in the hands is benign and does not require discontinuation of medication. Treatment: Low-dose propranolol, (10–30 mg tid) may be sufficient.

Hypothyroidism

Risks include female sex and tobacco use. Treatment: Thyroid supplementation.

Acne and Psoriasis

Common cause of patient-requested discontinuation of lithium. Treat as indicated.

Electroconvulsive Therapy

Electroconvulsive therapy (ECT) uses an electrical current to depolarize the brain, inducing a generalized seizure. ECT is used to treat a number of psychiatric illnesses and remains the most effective treatment for mood disorders. The mechanism of action is unclear, but ECT induces a number of changes in the brain, including changes in neurotransmitter and neuropeptide concentrations, changes in receptor density, activation of second messenger pathways, and induction of transcription. This appendix deals with the practical application of ECT in the treatment of psychiatric illness [1].

INDICATIONS

ECT is not generally used as a first-line treatment unless patients are unable to tolerate medical management of illness or the circumstances require rapid response of symptoms. Such situations may include malnutrition, catatonia, severe agitation, or suicidal behavior. ECT effectively treats mood symptoms, catatonia, and episodic psychotic symptoms. It is much less effective in the treatment of chronic psychotic symptoms or disorganization. The following are appropriate indications:

- Depression

- Mania

- Schizoaffaective disorder, particularly mood symptoms

- Acute psychosis in schizophrenia

- Catatonia

- Neuroleptic malignant syndrome

- Parkinson's disease

- Delirium

- Seizure disorders

CONTRAINDICATIONS

There are no absolute contraindications to ECT, including pregnancy and age limitations; however, there are relative contraindications and conditions that require special attention during the procedure. These fall into the categories of

- Cardiovascular conditions: recent infarction (MI), CAD, HTN, arrhythmia. ECT results in an immediate increase in parasympathetic tone that can precipitate bradyarrhythmias and asytole, followed by sympathetic release that increases BP and heart rate, placing high metabolic demands on the myocardium. It is thus advised that ECT not be given within 3 mos of an MI.

- Pulmonary conditions: COPD or asthma can affect oxygenation and should be treated with inhalers before ECT.

- Condition of the CNS: Brain tumor, aneurysm, recent intracerebral hemorrhage or infarction, and retinal detachment can be adversely impacted by increases in ICP and BP that occur during ECT.

- Conditions that increase risk for aspiration: GERD or even recent food. Patients should abstain from oral intake 8 hrs before treatment, and cricoid pressure should be applied during ECT for those at aspiration risk.

COMPLICATIONS

- Memory deficits: restricted to the time surrounding the procedure and are in excess of what might be anticipated for general anesthesia alone. Concomitant treatment with benzodiazepines or lithium, or bilateral electrode placement, may exacerbate acute cognitive deficits. Permanent deficits in learning have not been demonstrated.

- Myalgia: benign and self-limited.

- Headaches: Patients may be pretreated with NSAIDs.

- Cardiovascular complications: Asystole, tachyarrhythmias, and infarction are the usual causes of mortality.

- Cerebrovascular complications: Hemorrhagic stroke may occur secondary to increased BP.

- Regurgitation and aspiration: may result in aspiration pneumonitis.

- Death is rare (1:10,000 patients) and is usually due to cardiovascular complications.

WORKUP

- Complete psychiatric and physical evaluation focusing on risk factors for adverse outcomes

- CBC

- Electrolytes, BUN, creatinine

- ECG

- Chest x-ray

- Neuroimaging if papilledema or focal neurologic signs on exam

REFERENCE

1. Zorumski CF, Isenberg KE. Electroconvulsive therapy. In: Guze SB, ed. *Washington University adult psychiatry*. St. Louis: Mosby–Year Book, 1997:351–363.

D Orders and Notes

ADMISSION ORDERS

Date and time
Admit to (unit)
Legal status (voluntary, involuntary, voluntary by guardian)
Diagnosis (axis I–V)
Condition (satisfactory, guarded, critical)
Allergies (specify drug allergies)
Vitals (routine or specify protocol)
Activity and precautions (suicide, elopement, assault precautions,
   close observation with or without restrictions, one-on-one staffing,
   seclusion, restraints, etc.)
Nursing (if special staffing is required)
Diet (e.g., regular, MAOI diet, prudent diabetic, 1,800 cal ADA diet,
   Kosher meals)
IV (if necessary)
Labs (specify)
Meds (scheduled and prn)
Signature and name printed legibly

DISCHARGE ORDERS

Date and time
Discharge to (where—e.g., home, shelter, residential care) care of
   (whom—e.g., self, mother)
Diagnosis (axis I–V)
Condition on discharge (good, satisfactory)
Diet and activities
Meds (dosing instructions and amounts dispensed)
Follow-up arrangements
Signature and name printed legibly

ADMISSION NOTE

Date and time
Identifying information
Source of information
Chief complaint
History of present illness
Past medical history
Current meds
Drug allergies
Family psychiatric and medical history

Social and developmental history
Medical review of systems
Complete physical exam
Mental status exam
- General appearance and behavior
- Speech
- Thought process or flow
- Thought content
- Mood
- Affect
- Insight and judgment
- Sensorium and intellect

Assessment and plan: summary of the case, diagnoses on axis I–V, and treatment plan
Signature and name printed legibly

PROGRESS NOTE (EVALUATION AND MANAGEMENT):

Date and time
Subjective: includes interval history, patient's perspective on treatment progress, complaints of medication side effects, and subjective evaluation of symptoms.
Objective: current meds, vitals, lab results, nurses' charting (e.g., sleep, food intake), complete mental status exam.
Assessment: diagnosis on Axis I–V, interpretation of data in terms of treatment response and medication tolerance.
Plan: clinical decision making, medication changes, discharge planning, new studies ordered.
Signature and name printed legibly

DISCHARGE SUMMARY

Date and time
Date admitted
Date discharged
Identifying information
Presenting history
Mental status at presentation
Diagnostic labs and studies
Treatment and clinical course
Mental status at discharge
Discharge instructions
- Meds
- Activity
- Diet
- Follow-up arrangements

Condition on discharge
Signature and name printed legibly

Evaluating Clinical Outcome Studies

A clinician's prescribing practices are developed largely through experience; often, there are more treatment options available than there are data to support clinical decisions. Nonetheless, clinical outcome studies can play an important role in making decisions about which meds to prescribe in particular clinical situations. To fully benefit from the clinical literature, physicians must develop skills that allow them to critically evaluate published studies in terms of the design, validity, and applicability of the conclusions. Maintaining a rigorous critical mindset has become increasingly important as pharmaceutical industry sponsorship of continuing medical education and clinical trials becomes more pervasive. The following is a list of ten methodological errors that commonly lead to false conclusions in clinical trials.

1. **Making a big deal out of nothing.** Occurs when the makers of Drug X assert that it is equivalent to Drug Y based on the lack of a statistically significant difference in an underpowered comparison study. **Remember:** Statistical tests are designed to reject a null hypothesis (i.e., the "no difference" hypothesis), not to accept it.
2. **Implying clinical significance from statistical significance.** The makers of Drug X conduct a study using a large number of patients showing a statistically significant difference in weight gain between Drug X and Drug Y. The pharmaceutical sales representative reports that there is 3 times the weight gain with Drug Y, leading you to worry that your patients will become obese if you prescribe Drug Y. On examining the study, you realize that your concerns are excessive because the absolute magnitude of the weight gain difference is only 4 lb.
3. **Proof by meta-analysis.** Meta-analyses are used to compile data across multiple studies, thereby increasing statistical power to detect differences between groups. Meta-analyses are often subject to publication biases that favor positive results and should be evaluated cautiously along with the data from the included studies.
4. **Underdosing the active comparator.** The makers of Drug X assert that it is a better agent at controlling symptoms than Drug Y based on a study that compares Drug X to a subtherapeutic dose of Drug Y.
5. **Overdosing the active comparator.** The makers of Drug X assert that it has fewer side effects than Drug Y based on a study that compares Drug X to an unusually high dose of Drug Y.
6. **Comparing different sample populations.** The makers of Drug X claim that PO administration of Drug X controls psychotic

agitation as rapidly as IM injection of Drug Y. The claim is based on a study in which agitated patients were offered a choice between the two, and the ones who refused or were too agitated to respond received Drug Y. Thus, it seems likely that the more agitated and psychotic patients would be assigned to the group receiving Drug Y, making the comparison groups unequal.

7. **Using sensitive populations.** Conclusions about the superiority of the side effect profile of Drug X over Drug Y in all clinical situations are inferred from a study in which the comparison group is particularly sensitive to the side effect profile of Drug Y.

8. **Using specially selected populations.** The makers of Drug X claim that it is superior to Drug Y by showing greater efficacy in patients who have failed to respond to Drug Y. This claim is unfair, as the study does not compare efficacy in the general population but rather in a specially selected patient population (e.g., Drug Y nonresponders), which may be a very small proportion of the general population. Furthermore, Drug Y may show superiority to Drug X in a patient population that fails to respond to Drug X.

9. **Using measures with poor construct validity.** Often results obtained using standardized measurement tools can be contaminated by clinical factors that are not related to the clinical question being tested. For example, the presence of neuroleptic-induced parkinsonism artificially affects measures of depression or negative symptoms of schizophrenia because the hypokinesis and masked face can appear as psychomotor retardation or blunting of affect.

10. **Using adjunctive treatments unequally.** The makers of Drug X claim that there is no significant difference in the degree of anxiety or insomnia that it produces in comparison to drug Y. Review of the study reveals that the study allowed treatment with adjunctive benzodiazepines, and use of benzodiazepines was higher for the drug X comparison group, suggesting that Drug X is more anxiogenic.

F

DSM-IV
Diagnostic
Criteria*

DIAGNOSTIC CRITERIA FOR DELIRIUM DUE TO [INDICATE THE GENERAL MEDICAL CONDITION]

A. Disturbance of consciousness (i.e., reduced clarity of awareness of the environment) with reduced ability to focus, sustain, or shift attention.

B. A change in cognition (such as memory deficit, disorientation, language disturbance) or the development of a perceptual disturbance that is not better accounted for by a preexisting, established, or evolving dementia.

C. The disturbance develops over a short period of time (usually hours to days) and tends to fluctuate during the course of the day.

D. There is evidence from the history, physical examination, or laboratory findings that the disturbance is caused by the direct physiological consequences of a general medical condition.

DIAGNOSTIC CRITERIA FOR DEMENTIA OF THE ALZHEIMER'S TYPE

A. The development of multiple cognitive deficits manifested by both:
   (1) memory impairment (impaired ability to learn new information or to recall previously learned information)
   (2) one (or more) of the following cognitive disturbances:
      (a) aphasia (language disturbance)
      (b) apraxia (impaired ability to carry out motor activities despite intact motor function)
      (c) agnosia (failure to recognize or identify objects despite intact sensory function)
      (d) disturbance in executive functioning (i.e., planning, organizing, sequencing, abstracting)

B. The cognitive deficits in Criteria A1 and A2 each cause significant impairment in social or occupational functioning and represent a significant decline from a previous level of functioning.

C. The course is characterized by gradual onset and continuing cognitive decline.

D. The cognitive deficits in Criteria A1 and A2 are not due to any of the following:
   (1) other central nervous system conditions that cause progressive deficits in memory and cognition (e.g., cerebrovascular dis-

*Reprinted with permission from the *Diagnostic and statistical manual of mental disorders*, 4th ed. American Psychiatric Association, 1984.

ease, Parkinson's disease, Huntington's disease, subdural hematoma, normal-pressure hydrocephalus, brain tumor)

(2) systemic conditions that are known to cause dementia (e.g., hypothyroidism, vitamin B or folic acid deficiency, niacin deficiency, hypercalcemia, neurosyphilis, HIV infection)

(3) substance-induced conditions

E. The deficits do not occur exclusively during the course of a delirium.

F. The disturbance is not better accounted for by another Axis I disorder (e.g., Major Depressive Episode, Schizophrenia).

Text Revision. Copyright 2000, American Psychiatric Association.

DIAGNOSTIC CRITERIA FOR VASCULAR DEMENTIA

A. The development of multiple cognitive deficits manifested by both

(1) memory impairment (impaired ability to learn new information or to recall previously learned information)

(2) one (or more) of the following cognitive disturbances:

    (a) aphasia (language disturbance)

    (b) apraxia (impaired ability to carry out motor activities despite intact motor function)

    (c) agnosia (failure to recognize or identify objects despite intact sensory function)

    (d) disturbance in executive functioning (i.e., planning, organizing, sequencing, abstracting)

B. The cognitive deficits in Criteria A1 and A2 each cause significant impairment in social or occupational functioning and represent a significant decline from a previous level of functioning.

C. Focal neurological signs and symptoms (e.g., exaggeration of deep tendon reflexes, extensor plantar response, pseudobulbar palsy, gait abnormalities, weakness of an extremity) or laboratory evidence indicative of cerebrovascular disease (e.g., multiple infarctions involving cortex and underlying white matter) that are judged to be etiologically related to the disturbance.

D. The deficits do not occur exclusively during the course of a Delirium.

DIAGNOSTIC CRITERIA FOR SUBSTANCE ABUSE

A. A maladaptive pattern of substance use leading to clinically significant impairment or distress, as manifested by one (or more) of the following, occurring within a 12-month period:

(1) recurrent substance use resulting in a failure to fulfill major role obligations at work, school, or home (e.g., repeated absences or poor work performance related to substance use; substance-related absences, suspensions, or expulsions from school; neglect of children or household)

    (2) recurrent substance use in situations in which it is physically hazardous (e.g., driving an automobile or operating a machine when impaired by substance use)

    (3) recurrent substance-related legal problems (e.g., arrests for substance-related disorderly conduct)

    (4) continued substance use despite having persistent or recurrent social or interpersonal problems caused or exacerbated by the effects of the substance (e.g., arguments with spouse about consequences of Intoxication, physical fights)

B. The symptoms have never met the criteria for Substance Dependence for this class of substance.

DIAGNOSTIC CRITERIA FOR SUBSTANCE DEPENDENCE

A maladaptive pattern of substance use, leading to clinically significant impairment or distress, as manifested by three (or more) of the following, occurring at any time in the same 12-month period:

    (1) tolerance, as defined by either of the following:

        (a) a need for markedly increased amounts of the substance to achieve Intoxication or desired effect

        (b) markedly diminished effect with continued use of the same amount of the substance

    (2) withdrawal, as manifested by either of the following:

        (a) the characteristic withdrawal syndrome for the substance (refer to Criteria A and B of the criteria sets for Withdrawal from the specific substances)

        (b) the same (or a closely related) substance is taken to relieve or avoid withdrawal symptoms

    (3) the substance is often taken in larger amounts or over a longer period than was intended

    (4) there is a persistent desire or unsuccessful efforts to cut down or control substance use

    (5) a great deal of time is spent in activities necessary to obtain the substance (e.g., visiting multiple doctors or driving long distances), use the substance (e.g., chain-smoking), or recover from its effects

    (6) important social, occupational, or recreational activities are given up or reduced because of substance use

    (7) the substance use is continued despite knowledge of having a persistent or recurrent physical or psychological problem that is likely to have been caused or exacerbated by the substance (e.g., current cocaine use despite recognition of cocaine-induced depression, or continued drinking despite recognition that an ulcer was made worse by alcohol consumption)

Specify if:

With Physiological Dependence: evidence of tolerance or withdrawal (i.e., either Item 1 or 2 is present)

Without Physiological Dependence: no evidence of tolerance or withdrawal (i.e., neither Item 1 nor 2 is present)

DIAGNOSTIC CRITERIA FOR MAJOR DEPRESSIVE EPISODE

A. Five (or more) of the following symptoms have been present during the same 2-week period and represent a change from previous functioning; at least one of the symptoms is either (1) depressed mood or (2) loss of interest or pleasure. **Note:** Do not include symptoms that are clearly due to a general medical condition, or mood-incongruent delusions or hallucinations.

   (1) depressed mood most of the day, nearly every day, as indicated by either subjective report (e.g., feels sad or empty) or observation made by others (e.g., appears tearful). **Note:** In children and adolescents, can be irritable mood

   (2) markedly diminished interest or pleasure in all, or almost all, activities most of the day, nearly every day (as indicated by either subjective account or observation made by others)

   (3) significant weight loss when not dieting or weight gain (e.g., a change of more than 5% of body weight in a month), or decrease or increase in appetite nearly every day. **Note:** In children, consider failure to make expected weight gains

   (4) insomnia or hypersomnia nearly every day

   (5) psychomotor agitation or retardation nearly every day (observable by others, not merely subjective feelings of restlessness or being slowed down)

   (6) fatigue or loss of energy nearly every day

   (7) feelings of worthlessness or excessive or inappropriate guilt (which may be delusional) nearly every day (not merely self-reproach or guilt about being sick)

   (8) diminished ability to think or concentrate, or indecisiveness, nearly every day (either by subjective account or as observed by others)

   (9) recurrent thoughts of death (not just fear of dying), recurrent suicidal ideation without a specific plan, or a suicide attempt or a specific plan for committing suicide

B. The symptoms do not meet criteria for a Mixed Episode.

C. The symptoms cause clinically significant distress or impairment in social, occupational, or other important areas of functioning.

D. The symptoms are not due to the direct physiological effects of a substance (e.g., a drug of abuse, a medication) or a general medical condition (e.g., hypothyroidism).

E. The symptoms are not better accounted for by Bereavement—i.e., after the loss of a loved one, the symptoms persist for longer than 2 months or are characterized by marked functional impairment, morbid preoccupation with worthlessness, suicidal ideation, psychotic symptoms, or psychomotor retardation.

DIAGNOSTIC CRITERIA FOR A MANIC EPISODE

A. A distinct period of abnormally and persistently elevated, expansive, or irritable mood, lasting at least 1 week (or any duration if hospitalization is necessary).

B. During the period of mood disturbance, three (or more) of the following symptoms have persisted (four if the mood is only irritable) and have been present to a significant degree:

(1) inflated self-esteem or grandiosity

(2) decreased need for sleep (e.g., feels rested after only 3 hours of sleep)

(3) more talkative than usual or pressure to keep talking

(4) flight of ideas or subjective experience that thoughts are racing

(5) distractibility (i.e., attention too easily drawn to unimportant or irrelevant external stimuli)

(6) increase in goal-directed activity (either socially, at work or school, or sexually) or psychomotor agitation

(7) excessive involvement in pleasurable activities that have a high potential for painful consequences (e.g., engaging in unrestrained buying sprees, sexual indiscretions, or foolish business investments)

C. The symptoms do not meet criteria for a Mixed Episode.

D. The mood disturbance is sufficiently severe to cause marked impairment in occupational functioning or in usual social activities or relationships with others, or to necessitate hospitalization to prevent harm to self or others, or there are psychotic features.

E. The symptoms are not due to the direct physiological effects of a substance (e.g., a drug of abuse, a medication, or other treatment) or a general medical condition (e.g., hyperthyroidism).

DIAGNOSTIC CRITERIA FOR PANIC ATTACK

A discrete period of intense fear or discomfort, in which four (or more) of the following symptoms developed abruptly and reached a peak within 10 minutes:

1. palpitations, pounding heart, or accelerated heart rate
2. sweating
3. trembling or shaking
4. sensations of shortness of breath or smothering
5. feeling of choking
6. chest pain or discomfort
7. nausea or abdominal distress
8. feeling dizzy, unsteady, lightheaded, or faint
9. derealization (feelings of unreality) or depersonalization (being detached from oneself)
10. fear of losing control or going crazy
11. fear of dying
12. paresthesias (numbness or tingling sensations)
13. chills or hot flushes

DIAGNOSTIC CRITERIA FOR AGORAPHOBIA

A. Anxiety about being in places or situations from which escape might be difficult (or embarrassing) or in which help may not be available in the event of having an unexpected or situationally predisposed Panic Attack or panic-like symptoms. Agoraphobic fears typically involve characteristic clusters of situations that include being outside the home alone; being in a crowd or standing in a line; being on a bridge; and traveling in a bus, train, or automobile. **Note:** Consider the diagnosis of Specific Phobia if the avoidance is limited to one or only a few specific situations, or Social Phobia if the avoidance is limited to social situations.

B. The situations are avoided (e.g., travel is restricted) or else are endured with marked distress or with anxiety about having a Panic Attack or panic-like symptoms, or require the presence of a companion.

C. The anxiety or phobic avoidance is not better accounted for by another mental disorder, such as Social Phobia (e.g., avoidance limited to social situations because of fear of embarrassment), Specific Phobia (e.g., avoidance limited to a single situation like elevators), Obsessive-Compulsive Disorder (e.g., avoidance of dirt in someone with an obsession about contamination), Posttraumatic Stress Disorder (e.g., avoidance of stimuli associated with a severe stressor), or Separation Anxiety Disorder (e.g., avoidance of leaving home or relatives).

DIAGNOSTIC CRITERIA FOR SOCIAL PHOBIA

A. A marked and persistent fear of one or more social or performance situations in which the person is exposed to unfamiliar people or to possible scrutiny by others. The individual fears that he or she will act in a way (or show anxiety symptoms) that will be humiliating or embarrassing. **Note:** In children, there must be evidence of the capacity for age-appropriate social relationships with familiar people and the anxiety must occur in peer settings, not just in interactions with adults.

B. Exposure to the feared social situation almost invariably provokes anxiety, which may take the form of a situationally bound or situationally predisposed Panic Attack. **Note:** In children, the anxiety may be expressed by crying, tantrums, freezing, or shrinking from social situations with unfamiliar people.

C. The person recognizes that the fear is excessive or unreasonable. **Note:** In children, this feature may be absent.

D. The feared social or performance situations are avoided or else are endured with intense anxiety or distress.

E. The avoidance, anxious anticipation, or distress in the feared social or performance situation(s) interferes significantly with the person's normal routine, occupational (academic) functioning, or social activities or relationships, or there is marked distress about having the phobia.

F. In individuals under age 18 years, the duration is at least 6 months.

G. The fear or avoidance is not due to the direct physiological effects of a substance (e.g., a drug of abuse, a medication) or a general medical condition and is not better accounted for by another mental disorder (e.g., Panic Disorder with or without Agoraphobia, Separation Anxiety Disorder, Body Dysmorphic Disorder, a Pervasive Developmental Disorder, or Schizoid Personality Disorder).

H. If a general medical condition or another mental disorder is present, the fear in Criterion A is unrelated to it—e.g., the fear is not of Stuttering, trembling in Parkinson's disease, or exhibiting abnormal eating behavior in Anorexia Nervosa or Bulimia Nervosa.

DIAGNOSTIC CRITERIA FOR OBSESSIVE-COMPULSIVE DISORDER

A. Either obsessions or compulsions:
Obsessions as defined by (1), (2), (3), and (4):

(1) recurrent and persistent thoughts, impulses, or images that are experienced, at some time during the disturbance, as intrusive and inappropriate and that cause marked anxiety or distress

(2) the thoughts, impulses, or images are not simply excessive worries about real-life problems

(3) the person attempts to ignore or suppress such thoughts, impulses, or images, or to neutralize them with some other thought or action

(4) the person recognizes that the obsessional thoughts, impulses, or images are a product of his or her own mind (not imposed from without as in thought insertion)

Compulsions as defined by (1) and (2):

(1) repetitive behaviors (e.g., hand washing, ordering, checking) or mental acts (e.g., praying, counting, repeating words silently) that the person feels driven to perform in response to an obsession, or according to rules that must be applied rigidly

(2) the behaviors or mental acts are aimed at preventing or reducing distress or preventing some dreaded event or situation; however, these behaviors or mental acts either are not connected in a realistic way with what they are designed to neutralize or prevent or are clearly excessive

B. At some point during the course of the disorder, the person has recognized that the obsessions or compulsions are excessive or unreasonable. **Note:** This does not apply to children.

C. The obsessions or compulsions cause marked distress, are time consuming (take more than 1 hour a day), or significantly interfere with the person's normal routine, occupational (or academic) functioning, or usual social activities or relationships.

D. If another Axis I disorder is present, the content of the obsessions or compulsions is not restricted to it (e.g., preoccupation with food in the presence of an Eating Disorder; hair pulling in the presence of Trichotillomania; concern with appearance in the presence of Body Dysmorphic Disorder; preoccupation with drugs in the presence of a Substance Use Disorder; preoccupation with having a serious illness in the presence of Hypochondriasis; preoccupation with sexual urges or fantasies in the presence of a Paraphilia; or guilty ruminations in the presence of Major Depressive Disorder).

E. The disturbance is not due to the direct physiological effects of a substance (e.g., a drug of abuse, a medication) or a general medical condition.

DIAGNOSTIC CRITERIA FOR POSTTRAUMATIC STRESS DISORDER

A. The person has been exposed to a traumatic event in which both of the following were present:

  (1) the person experienced, witnessed, or was confronted with an event or events that involved actual or threatened death or serious injury, or a threat to the physical integrity of self or others

  (2) the person's response involved intense fear, helplessness, or horror. **Note:** In children, this may be expressed instead by disorganized or agitated behavior

B. The traumatic event is persistently reexperienced in one (or more) of the following ways:

  (1) recurrent and intrusive distressing recollections of the event, including images, thoughts, or perceptions. **Note:** In young children, repetitive play may occur in which themes or aspects of the trauma are expressed.

  (2) recurrent distressing dreams of the event. **Note:** In children, there may be frightening dreams without recognizable content.

  (3) acting or feeling as if the traumatic event were recurring (includes a sense of reliving the experience, illusions, hallucinations, and dissociative flashback episodes, including those that occur on awakening or when intoxicated). **Note:** In young children, trauma-specific reenactment may occur.

  (4) intense psychological distress at exposure to internal or external cues that symbolize or resemble an aspect of the traumatic event

  (5) physiological reactivity on exposure to internal or external cues that symbolize or resemble an aspect of the traumatic event

C. Persistent avoidance of stimuli associated with the trauma and numbing of general responsiveness (not present before the trauma), as indicated by three (or more) of the following:

  (1) efforts to avoid thoughts, feelings, or conversations associated with the trauma

  (2) efforts to avoid activities, places, or people that arouse recollections of the trauma

  (3) inability to recall an important aspect of the trauma

  (4) markedly diminished interest or participation in significant activities

(5) feeling of detachment or estrangement from others

(6) restricted range of affect (e.g., unable to have loving feelings)

(7) sense of a foreshortened future (e.g., does not expect to have a career, marriage, children, or a normal life span)

D. Persistent symptoms of increased arousal (not present before the trauma), as indicated by two (or more) of the following:

(1) difficulty falling or staying asleep

(2) irritability or outbursts of anger

(3) difficulty concentrating

(4) hypervigilance

(5) exaggerated startle response

E. Duration of the disturbance (symptoms in Criteria B, C, and D) is more than 1 month.

F. The disturbance causes clinically significant distress or impairment in social, occupational, or other important areas of functioning.

DIAGNOSTIC CRITERIA FOR GENERALIZED ANXIETY DISORDER

A. Excessive anxiety and worry (apprehensive expectation), occurring more days than not for at least 6 months, about a number of events or activities (such as work or school performance).

B. The person finds it difficult to control the worry.

C. The anxiety and worry are associated with three (or more) of the following six symptoms (with at least some symptoms present for more days than not for the past 6 months). **Note:** Only one item is required in children.

(1) restlessness or feeling keyed up or on edge

(2) being easily fatigued

(3) difficulty concentrating or mind going blank

(4) irritability

(5) muscle tension

(6) sleep disturbance (difficulty falling or staying asleep, or restless unsatisfying sleep)

D. The focus of the anxiety and worry is not confined to features of an Axis I disorder—e.g., the anxiety or worry is not about having a Panic Attack (as in Panic Disorder), being embarrassed in public (as in Social Phobia), being contaminated (as in Obsessive-Compulsive Disorder), being away from home or close relatives (as in Separation Anxiety Disorder), gaining weight (as in Anorexia Nervosa), having multiple physical complaints (as in Somatization Disorder), or having a serious illness (as in Hypochondriasis), and the anxiety and worry do not occur exclusively during Posttraumatic Stress Disorder.

E. The anxiety, worry, or physical symptoms cause clinically significant distress or impairment in social, occupational, or other important areas of functioning.

F. The disturbance is not due to the direct physiological effects of a substance (e.g., a drug of abuse, a medication) or a general medical condition (e.g., hyperthyroidism) and does not occur exclusively during a Mood Disorder, a Psychotic Disorder, or a Pervasive Developmental Disorder.

DIAGNOSTIC CRITERIA FOR SCHIZOPHRENIA

A. Characteristic symptoms: Two (or more) of the following, each present for a significant portion of time during a 1-month period (or less if successfully treated):

(1) delusions
(2) hallucinations
(3) disorganized speech (e.g., frequent derailment or incoherence)
(4) grossly disorganized or catatonic behavior
(5) negative symptoms—i.e., affective flattening, alogia, or avolition

Note: Only one Criterion A symptom is required if delusions are bizarre or hallucinations consist of a voice keeping up a running commentary on the person's behavior or thoughts, or two or more voices conversing with each other.

B. Social/occupational dysfunction: For a significant portion of the time since the onset of the disturbance, one or more major areas of functioning such as work, interpersonal relations, or self-care are markedly below the level achieved prior to the onset (or when the onset is in childhood or adolescence, failure to achieve expected level of interpersonal, academic, or occupational achievement).

C. Duration: Continuous signs of the disturbance persist for at least 6 months. This 6-month period must include at least 1 month of symptoms (or less if successfully treated) that meet Criterion A (i.e., active-phase symptoms) and may include periods of prodromal or residual symptoms. During these prodromal or residual periods, the signs of the disturbance may be manifested by only negative symptoms or two or more symptoms listed in Criterion A present in an attenuated form (e.g., odd beliefs, unusual perceptual experiences).

D. Schizoaffective and Mood Disorder exclusion: Schizoaffective Disorder and Mood Disorder With Psychotic Features have been ruled out because either (1) no Major Depressive, Manic, or Mixed Episodes have occurred concurrently with the active-phase symptoms; or (2) if mood episodes have occurred during active-phase symptoms, their total duration has been brief relative to the duration of the active and residual periods.

E. Substance/general medical condition exclusion: The disturbance is not due to the direct physiological effects of a substance (e.g., a drug of abuse, a medication) or a general medical condition.

F. Relationship to a Pervasive Developmental Disorder: If there is a history of Autistic Disorder or another Pervasive Developmental Disorder, the additional diagnosis of Schizophrenia is made only if prominent delusions or hallucinations are also present for at least a month (or less if successfully treated).

DIAGNOSTIC CRITERIA FOR (SCHIZOPHRENIA) CATATONIC TYPE

A. A type of Schizophrenia in which the clinical picture is dominated by at least two of the following:
   (1) motoric immobility as evidenced by catalepsy (including waxy flexibility) or stupor
   (2) excessive motor activity (that is apparently purposeless and not influenced by external stimuli)
   (3) extreme negativism (an apparently motiveless resistance to all instructions or maintenance of a rigid posture against attempts to be moved) or mutism
   (4) peculiarities of voluntary movement as evidenced by posturing (voluntary assumption of inappropriate or bizarre postures), stereotyped movements, prominent mannerisms, or prominent grimacing
   (5) echolalia or echopraxia

DIAGNOSTIC CRITERIA FOR SCHIZOAFFECTIVE DISORDER

A. An uninterrupted period of illness during which, at some time, there is either a Major Depressive Episode, a Manic Episode, or a Mixed Episode concurrent with symptoms that meet Criterion A for Schizophrenia. **Note:** The Major Depressive Episode must include Criterion A1: depressed mood.

B. During the same period of illness, there have been delusions or hallucinations for at least 2 weeks in the absence of prominent mood symptoms.

C. Symptoms that meet criteria for a mood episode are present for a substantial portion of the total duration of the active and residual periods of the illness.

D. The disturbance is not due to the direct physiological effects of a substance (e.g., a drug of abuse, a medication) or a general medical condition.

Specify type:

   Bipolar Type: if the disturbance includes a Manic or a Mixed Episode (or a Manic or a Mixed Episode and Major Depressive Episodes)

   Depressive Type: if the disturbance only includes Major Depressive Episodes

DIAGNOSTIC CRITERIA FOR SOMATIZATION DISORDER

A. A history of many physical complaints beginning before age 30 years that occur over a period of several years and result in treatment being sought or significant impairment in social, occupational, or other important areas of functioning.

B. Each of the following criteria must have been met, with individual symptoms occurring at any time during the course of the disturbance:

(1) four pain symptoms: a history of pain related to at least four different sites or functions (e.g., head, abdomen, back, joints, extremities, chest, rectum, during menstruation, during sexual intercourse, or during urination)

(2) two gastrointestinal symptoms: a history of at least two gastrointestinal symptoms other than pain (e.g., nausea, bloating, vomiting other than during pregnancy, diarrhea, or intolerance of several different foods)

(3) one sexual symptom: a history of at least one sexual or reproductive symptom other than pain (e.g., sexual indifference, erectile or ejaculatory dysfunction, irregular menses, excessive menstrual bleeding, vomiting throughout pregnancy)

(4) one pseudoneurological symptom: a history of at least one symptom or deficit suggesting a neurological condition not limited to pain (conversion symptoms such as impaired coordination or balance, paralysis or localized weakness, difficulty swallowing or lump in throat, aphonia, urinary retention, hallucinations, loss of touch or pain sensation, double vision, blindness, deafness, seizures; dissociative symptoms such as amnesia; or loss of consciousness other than fainting)

C. Either (1) or (2):

(1) after appropriate investigation, each of the symptoms in Criterion B cannot be fully explained by a known general medical condition or the direct effects of a substance (e.g., a drug of abuse, a medication)

(2) when there is a related general medical condition, the physical complaints or resulting social or occupational impairment are in excess of what would be expected from the history, physical examination, or laboratory findings

D. The symptoms are not intentionally feigned or produced (as in Factitious Disorder or Malingering).

DIAGNOSTIC CRITERIA FOR FACTITIOUS DISORDER

A. Intentional production or feigning of physical or psychological signs or symptoms.

B. The motivation for the behavior is to assume the sick role.

C. External incentives for the behavior (such as economic gain, avoiding legal responsibility, or improving physical well-being, as in Malingering) are absent.

Code based on type:

With Predominantly Psychological Signs and Symptoms: if psychological signs and symptoms predominate in the clinical presentation

With Predominantly Physical Signs and Symptoms: if physical signs and symptoms predominate in the clinical presentation

With Combined Psychological and Physical Signs and Symptoms: if both psychological and physical signs and symptoms are present but neither predominates in the clinical presentation

GENERAL DIAGNOSTIC CRITERIA FOR A PERSONALITY DISORDER

A. An enduring pattern of inner experience and behavior that deviates markedly from the expectations of the individual's culture. This pattern is manifested in two (or more) of the following areas:
   (1) cognition (i.e., ways of perceiving and interpreting self, other people, and events)
   (2) affectivity (i.e., the range, intensity, lability, and appropriateness of emotional response)
   (3) interpersonal functioning
   (4) impulse control

B. The enduring pattern is inflexible and pervasive across a broad range of personal and social situations.

C. The enduring pattern leads to clinically significant distress or impairment in social, occupational, or other important areas of functioning.

D. The pattern is stable and of long duration and its onset can be traced back at least to adolescence or early adulthood.

E. The enduring pattern is not better accounted for as a manifestation or consequence of another mental disorder.

F. The enduring pattern is not due to the direct physiological effects of a substance (e.g., a drug of abuse, a medication) or a general medical condition (e.g., head trauma).

Text Revision. Copyright 2000, American Psychiatric Association.

DIAGNOSTIC CRITERIA FOR CONDUCT DISORDER

A. A repetitive and persistent pattern of behavior in which the basic rights of others or major age-appropriate societal norms or rules are violated, as manifested by the presence of three (or more) of the following criteria in the past 12 months, with at least one criterion present in the past 6 months:

Aggression to people and animals
   (1) often bullies, threatens, or intimidates others
   (2) often initiates physical fights
   (3) has used a weapon that can cause serious physical harm to others (e.g., bat, brick, broken bottle, knife, gun)
   (4) has been physically cruel to people
   (5) has been physically cruel to animals
   (6) has stolen while confronting a victim (e.g., mugging, purse snatching, extortion, armed robbery)
   (7) has forced someone into sexual activity

Destruction of property
   (8) has deliberately engaged in fire setting with the intention of causing serious damage
   (9) has deliberately destroyed others' property (other than by fire setting)

Deceitfulness or theft
   (10) has broken into someone else's house, building, or car

(11) often lies to obtain goods or favors or to avoid obligations (i.e., "cons" others)

(12) has stolen items of nontrivial value without confronting a victim (e.g., shoplifting, but without breaking and entering; forgery)

Serious violations of rules

(13) often stays out at night despite parental prohibitions, beginning before age 13 years

(14) has run away from home overnight at least twice while living in parental or parental surrogate home (or once without returning for a lengthy period)

(15) is often truant from school, beginning before age 13 years

B. The disturbance in behavior causes clinically significant impairment in social, academic, or occupational functioning.

C. If the individual is age 18 years or older, criteria are not met for Antisocial Personality Disorder.

DIAGNOSTIC CRITERIA FOR ANTISOCIAL PERSONALITY DISORDER

A. There is a pervasive pattern of disregard for and violation of the rights of others occurring since age 15 years, as indicated by three (or more) of the following:

(1) failure to conform to social norms with respect to lawful behaviors as indicated by repeatedly performing acts that are grounds for arrest

(2) deceitfulness, as indicated by repeated lying, use of aliases, or conning others for personal profit or pleasure

(3) impulsivity or failure to plan ahead

(4) irritability and aggressiveness, as indicated by repeated physical fights or assaults

(5) reckless disregard for safety of self or others

(6) consistent irresponsibility, as indicated by repeated failure to sustain consistent work behavior or honor financial obligations

(7) lack of remorse, as indicated by being indifferent to or rationalizing having hurt, mistreated, or stolen from another

B. The individual is at least age 18 years.

C. There is evidence of Conduct Disorder with onset before age 15 years.

D. The occurrence of antisocial behavior is not exclusively during the course of Schizophrenia or a Manic Episode.

DIAGNOSTIC CRITERIA FOR BORDERLINE PERSONALITY DISORDER

A pervasive pattern of instability of interpersonal relationships, self-image, and affects, and marked impulsivity beginning by early adulthood and present in a variety of contexts, as indicated by five (or more) of the following:

(1) frantic efforts to avoid real or imagined abandonment. **Note:** Do not include suicidal or self-mutilating behavior covered in Criterion 5.
(2) a pattern of unstable and intense interpersonal relationships characterized by alternating between extremes of idealization and devaluation
(3) identity disturbance: markedly and persistently unstable self-image or sense of self
(4) impulsivity in at least two areas that are potentially self-damaging (e.g., spending, sex, Substance Abuse, reckless driving, binge eating). **Note:** Do not include suicidal or self-mutilating behavior covered in Criterion 5.
(5) recurrent suicidal behavior, gestures, or threats, or self-mutilating behavior
(6) affective instability due to a marked reactivity of mood (e.g., intense episodic dysphoria, irritability, or anxiety usually lasting a few hours and only rarely more than a few days)
(7) chronic feelings of emptiness
(8) inappropriate, intense anger or difficulty controlling anger (e.g., frequent displays of temper, constant anger, recurrent physical fights)
(9) transient, stress-related paranoid ideation or severe dissociative symptoms

G

Standardized Assessment Tools

FOLSTEIN MINI MENTAL STATUS EXAM

Skill	Test	Scoring	Total points
Orientation, time	What is the date?	Score 1 point each for year, season, date, month, and day of the week.	5
Orientation, place	Where are you?	Score 1 point each for state, county, city, building, and floor.	5
Immediate recall/ repetition	I'm going to name three objects, and I want you to repeat them. Remember what they are because I will be asking you to recall them in about 5 minutes. Dog, car, ball.	Score 1 point for each item repeated. If the patient fails to register all three, repeat them until the patient is successful.	3
Concentration	Can you spell the word "world"? Spell "world" backward.	Score 1 point for each correct answer backward. Patient must be able to spell "world" forward in order to correctly evaluate backward performance. An alternative test is to ask the patient to say the months of the year backward from December.	5
Naming	Point to your pen and ask the patient "What is this called?" Repeat with watch or belt.	Score 1 point for each object named.	2
Repetition	Say "no ifs, ands, or buts."	Score 1 point if repeated correctly on the first try.	1
Short-term recall	What were those three words I asked you to remember earlier?	Score 1 point for each item recalled.	3
Verbal commands	Grab your left ear with your right hand.	Score 1 point for grabbing the right ear with the right hand or left ear with the left hand, two points for crossing the midline, and three points for correct performance.	3

(continued)

FOLSTEIN MINI MENTAL STATUS EXAM (continued)

Skill	Test	Scoring	Total points
Written commands	I'm going to test your ability to follow written commands. Show the patient a piece of paper with the words "CLOSE YOUR EYES" written on it.	Score 1 point if the patient closes his eyes.	1
Writing	Write a sentence.	Score 1 point if the sentence is grammatically correct.	1
Drawing	Draw a clock.	Score 1 point if the clock has two hands and the numbers are correctly placed.	1

Adapted from Folstein MF, Folstein SE, McHugh PR. "Mini-mental state." A practical method for grading the cognitive state of patients for the clinician. *J Psychiatr Res* 1975;12:189–198.

HAMILTON RATING SCALE FOR DEPRESSION

For each item select the "cue" which best characterizes the patient.

1: Depressed mood (sadness, hopeless, helpless, worthless)
  0 Absent
  1 These feeling states indicated only on questioning
  2 These feeling states spontaneously reported verbally
  3 Communicates feeling states nonverbally—i.e., through facial expression, posture, voice, and tendency to weep
  4 Patient reports VIRTUALLY ONLY these feeling states in his spontaneous verbal and nonverbal communication

2: Feelings of guilt
  0 Absent
  1 Self-reproach, feels he has let people down
  2 Ideas of guilt or rumination over past errors or sinful deeds
  3 Present illness is a punishment. Delusions of guilt
  4 Hears accusatory or denunciatory voices and/or experiences threatening visual hallucinations

3: Suicide
  0 Absent
  1 Feels life is not worth living
  2 Wishes he were dead or any thoughts of possible death to self
  3 Suicide ideas or gesture
  4 Attempts at suicide (any serious attempt rates 4)

4: Insomnia early
  0 No difficulty falling asleep
  1 Complains of occasional difficulty falling asleep—i.e., more than $1/4$ hour
  2 Complains of nightly difficulty falling asleep

5: Insomnia middle
  0 No difficulty
  1 Patient complains of being restless and disturbed during the night
  2 Waking during the night—any getting out of bed rates 2 (except for purpose of voiding)

6: Insomnia late
  0 No difficulty
  1 Waking in early hours of the morning but goes back to sleep
  2 Unable to fall asleep again if gets out of bed

7: Work and activities
  0 No difficulty
  1 Thoughts and feelings of incapacity, fatigue, or weakness related to activities, work, or hobbies
  2 Loss of interest in activity, hobbies, or work—either directly reported by patient, or indirect in listlessness, indecision, and vacillation (feels he has to push self to work or activities)
  3 Decrease in actual time spent in activities or decrease in productivity. In hospital, rate 3 if patient does not spend at least three hours a day in activities (hospital job or hobbies) exclusive of ward chores
  4 Stopped working because of present illness. In hospital, rate 4 if patient engages in no activities except ward chores, or if patient fails to perform ward chores unassisted

8: Retardation (slowness of thought and speech; impaired ability to concentrate; decreased motor activity)

(continued)

HAMILTON RATING SCALE FOR DEPRESSION (*continued*)

- 0 Normal speech and thought
- 1 Slight retardation at interview
- 2 Obvious retardation at interview
- 3 Interview difficult
- 4 Complete stupor

9: Agitation
- 0 None
- 1 "Playing with" hands, hair, etc.
- 2 Hand-wringing, nail biting, hair pulling, biting of lips

10: Anxiety psychic
- 0 No difficulty
- 1 Subjective tension and irritability
- 2 Worrying about minor matters
- 3 Apprehensive attitude apparent in face or speech
- 4 Fears expressed without questioning

11: Anxiety somatic
- 0 Absent
- 1 Mild
- 2 Moderate
- 3 Severe
- 4 Incapacitating

Physiological concomitants of anxiety, such as:

Gastrointestinal—dry mouth, wind, indigestion, diarrhea, cramps, belching
Cardiovascular—palpitations, headaches
Respiratory—hyperventilation, sighing
Urinary frequency
Sweating

12: Somatic symptoms gastrointestinal
- 0 None
- 1 Loss of appetite but eating without staff encouragement. Heavy feelings in abdomen.
- 2. Difficulty eating without staff urging; requests or requires laxatives or medication for bowels or medication for GI symptoms

13: Somatic symptoms general
- 0 None
- 1 Heaviness in limbs, back or head. Backaches, headache, muscle aches. Loss of energy and fatigability.
- 2 Any clear-cut symptom rates 2

14: Genital symptoms
- 0 Absent
- 1 Mild
- 2 Severe

Symptoms such as:

Loss of libido
Menstrual disturbances

15: Hypochondriasis
- 0 Not present
- 1 Self-absorption (bodily)

(*continued*)

HAMILTON RATING SCALE FOR DEPRESSION
(*continued*)

    2 Preoccupation with health
    3 Frequent complaints, requests for help, etc.
    4 Hypochondriacal delusions
16: Loss of weight
    A: When rating by history
        0 No weight loss
        1 Probable weight loss associated with present illness
        2 Definite (according to patient) weight loss
    B: On weekly ratings by ward psychiatrist, when actual weight changes
       are measured
        0 Less than 1-lb weight loss in week
        1 Greater than 1-lb weight loss in week
        2 Greater than 2-lb weight loss in week
17: Insight
    0 Acknowledges being depressed and ill
    1 Acknowledges illness but attributes cause to bad food, climate, over-
      work, virus, need for rest, etc.
    2 Denies being ill at all
18: Diurnal variation
   a.m. p.m.
    0   0   Absent
    1   1   Mild
    2   2   Severe
If symptoms are worse in the morning or evening, note which it is and rate severity of variation
19: Depersonalization and derealization
    0 Absent
    1 Mild
    2 Moderate
    3 Severe
    4 Incapacitating
Such as:
    Feeling of unreality
    Nihilistic ideas
20: Paranoid symptoms
    0 None
    1,2 Suspiciousness
    3 Ideas of reference
    4 Delusions of reference and persecution
21: Obsessional and compulsive symptoms
    0 Absent
    1 Mild
    2 Severe
22: Helplessness
    0 Not present
    1 Subjective feelings which are elicited only by inquiry
    2 Patient volunteers his helpless feelings
    3 Requires urging, guidance, and reassurance to accomplish ward chores or
      personal hygiene

(*continued*)

HAMILTON RATING SCALE FOR DEPRESSION (*continued*)

  4 Requires physical assistance for dress, grooming, eating, bedside tasks, or personal hygiene
23: Hopelessness
  0 Not present
  1 Intermittently doubts that "things will improve" but can be reassured
  2 Consistently feels "hopeless" but accepts reassurances
  3 Expresses feelings of discouragement, despair, pessimism about future, which cannot be dispelled
  4 Spontaneously and inappropriately perseverates: "I'll never get well" or its equivalent
24: Worthlessness (ranges from mild loss of esteem, feelings of inferiority, self-deprecation to delusional notions of worthlessness)
  0 Not present
  1 Indicates feelings of worthlessness (loss of self-esteem) only on questioning
  2 Spontaneously indicates feelings of worthlessness (loss of self-esteem)
  3 Different from 2 by degree. Patient volunteers that he is "no good," "inferior," etc.
  4 Delusional notions of worthlessness—i.e., "I am a heap of garbage" or its equivalent

Reprinted with permission from Hamilton M. A rating scale for depression. *J Neurol Neurosurg Psychiatry* 1960;23:56.

BRIEF PSYCHIATRIC RATING SCALE

Directions: Place an X in the appropriate box to represent the level of severity of each symptom.

Patient_____

Rater_____

No._____

Date_____

	Not present = 0	Very mild = 1	Mild = 2	Moderate = 3	Mod. severe = 4	Severe = 5	Extremely severe = 6
	0	1	2	3	4	5	6
1. Somatic concern—preoccupation with physical health, fear of physical illness, hypochondriases	❑	❑	❑	❑	❑	❑	❑
2. Anxiety—worry, fear, overconcern for present or future	❑	❑	❑	❑	❑	❑	❑
3. Emotional withdrawal—lack of spontaneous interaction, isolation, deficiency in relating to others	❑	❑	❑	❑	❑	❑	❑
4. Conceptual disorganization—thought processes confused, disconnected, disorganized, disrupted	❑	❑	❑	❑	❑	❑	❑
5. Guilt feelings—self-blame, shame, remorse for past behavior	❑	❑	❑	❑	❑	❑	❑
6. Tension—physical and motor manifestations or nervousness, overactivation, tension	❑	❑	❑	❑	❑	❑	❑
7. Mannerisms and posturing—peculiar, bizarre, unnatural motor behavior (not including tic)	❑	❑	❑	❑	❑	❑	❑
8. Grandiosity—exaggerated self-opinion, arrogance, conviction of unusual power or abilities	❑	❑	❑	❑	❑	❑	❑
9. Depressive mood—sorrow, sadness, despondency, pessimism	❑	❑	❑	❑	❑	❑	❑

	Not present = 0	Very mild = 1	Mild = 2	Moderate = 3	Mod. severe = 4	Severe = 5	Extremely severe = 6
	0	1	2	3	4	5	6
10. Hostility—animosity, contempt, belligerence, disdain for others	❑	❑	❑	❑	❑	❑	❑
11. Suspiciousness—mistrust, belief that others harbor malicious or discriminatory intent	❑	❑	❑	❑	❑	❑	❑
12. Hallucinatory behavior—perceptions without normal external stimulus correspondence	❑	❑	❑	❑	❑	❑	❑
13. Motor retardation—slowed, weakened movements or speech, reduced body tone	❑	❑	❑	❑	❑	❑	❑
14. Uncooperativeness—resistance, guardedness, rejection of authority	❑	❑	❑	❑	❑	❑	❑
15. Unusual thought content—unusual, odd, strange, bizarre thought content	❑	❑	❑	❑	❑	❑	❑
16. Blunted affect—reduced emotional tone, reduction in normal intensity of feelings, flatness	❑	❑	❑	❑	❑	❑	❑
17. Excitement—heightened emotional tone, agitation, increased reactivity	❑	❑	❑	❑	❑	❑	❑
18. Disorientation, confusion or lack of proper association for person, place, or time	❑	❑	❑	❑	❑	❑	❑

From Overall JE, Gorham DR. The brief psychiatric rating scale. *Psychol Rep* 1962;10:799–812. © Southern Universities Press, 1962.

ABNORMAL INVOLUNTARY MOVEMENT SCALE (AIMS) EXAMINATION PROCEDURE

Patient identification: _____ Date: _____

Rated by: _____

Either before or after completing the examination procedure, observe the patient unobtrusively at rest (e.g., in waiting room).

The chair to be used in this examination should be a hard, firm one without arms.

After observing the patient, he or she may be rated on a scale of 0 (none), 1 (minimal), 2 (mild), 3 (moderate), and 4 (severe) according to the severity of symptoms.

Ask the patient whether there is anything in his/her mouth (i.e., gum, candy, etc.) and if there is to remove it.

Ask patient about the current condition of his/her teeth. Ask patient if he/she wears dentures. Do teeth or dentures bother patient now?

Ask patient whether he/she notices any movement in mouth, face, hands, or feet. If yes, ask to describe and to what extent they currently bother patient or interfere with his/her activities.

0 1 2 3 4	Have patient sit in chair with hands on knees, legs slightly apart, and feet flat on floor. (Look at entire body for movements while in this position.)
0 1 2 3 4	Ask patient to sit with hands hanging unsupported. If male, between legs; if female and wearing a dress, hanging over knees. (Observe hands and other body areas.)
0 1 2 3 4	Ask patient to open mouth. (Observe tongue at rest within mouth.) Do this twice.
0 1 2 3 4	Ask patient to protrude tongue. (Observe abnormalities of tongue movement.) Do this twice.
0 1 2 3 4	Ask the patient to tap thumb, with each finger, as rapidly as possible for 10–15 seconds; separately with right hand, then with left hand. (Observe facial and leg movements.)
0 1 2 3 4	Flex and extend patient's left and right arms. (One at a time.)
0 1 2 3 4	Ask patient to stand up. (Observe in profile. Observe all body areas again, hips included.)
0 1 2 3 4	Ask patient to extend both arms outstretched in front with palms down. (Observe trunk, legs, and mouth.)[a]
0 1 2 3 4	Have patient walk a few paces, turn, and walk back to chair. (Observe hands and gait.) Do this twice.[a]

[a]Activated movements.

Patient Data
Tracking Form

Date: _____ Time: _____

Axis I: _____
Axis II: _____ **Axis IV:** _____
Axis III: _____ **Axis V:** _____

Sources of info: The patient, who appears ❑ Reliable ❑ Largely reliable
  ❑ Unreliable _____
  ❑ Medical record ❑ Other (specify) _____

ID info: ❑ Voluntary ❑ Involuntary _____
_____

Chief complaint: _____

History of present illness: _____
_____
_____
_____
_____

History of ❑ Mania ❑ Psychosis ❑ Depression ❑ Suicide attempts
  ❑ Hospitalization ❑ Treatment _____

Past medical/surgical history: _____
_____
_____

Allergies: ❑ NKDA _____

Medications: _____
_____

Social history: ❑ Childhood/youth _____
  ❑ Single ❑ Married ❑ Divorced ❑ Widowed Living situation: _____
Children: _____
Occupational history: _____
Legal history: _____
❑ No alcohol ❑ Alcohol in past ❑ Drinks: _____
❑ Does not smoke ❑ Smoked in past ❑ Smokes: _____
❑ No recreational drugs ❑ Cocaine: _____ ❑ Marijuana: _____
❑ Heroin: _____ ❑ Other: _____

Assets: _____

Family history:
Depression: _____ Alcoholism: _____
Bipolar disorder: _____ Drug use: _____
Schizophrenia/Psychoses: _____ Suicide: _____

Dementia: _____ Other: _____

Review of systems:

HEENT: ❑ Headache ❑ Dizziness ❑ Fatigue ❑ Blurred vision ❑ Diplopia
❑ Hearing problems ❑ Tinnitus ❑ Vertigo ❑ Sore throat ❑ Hoarseness
❑ Trouble swallowing ❑ Other _____

CV: ❑ Chest pain/discomfort ❑ Palpitations ❑ Leg swelling ❑ Other: _____
RESP: ❑ Dyspnea ❑ Tachypnea ❑ Cough ❑ Other: _____
GI: ❑ Nausea ❑ Vomiting ❑ Abdominal pain ❑ Diarrhea ❑ Constipation
❑ Other: _____
GU: ❑ Dysuria ❑ Urgency ❑ Incontinence ❑ Irregular menses
❑ Other _____

OTHER: ❑ Joint pain ❑ Myalgia ❑ Pruritis ❑ Other

❑ ALL OTHER SYSTEMS ARE NEGATIVE

Physical exam:

T____ HR ____ RR ____ BP ____

HEENT:
❑ Head atraumatic ❑ White sclera ❑ No bruits
❑ Moist membranes ❑ No thyro ❑ No lymph
CARDIO/PULMONARY:
❑ Normal R&R ❑ No MRG ❑ Lungs CTA
ABDOMEN:
❑ NTND ❑ No hepatosplenomegaly ❑ Normal BS

EXTREMITIES:

❑ No scars ❑ No edema ❑ Palpable pulses

NEUROLOGIC:

❑ PERLL ❑ EOMI ❑ Visual acuity/fields intact
❑ Face symmetric ❑ Facial sensation intact
❑ Hearing intact ❑ Palate rises symmetrically
❑ Shoulder shrug equal ❑ Tongue midline
❑ Motor tone normal ❑ Motor strength 5/5
❑ Sensation grossly intact ❑ DTRs 2/5
❑ Coordination intact ❑ Posture/gait normal

Labs/Tests:

Mental Status Exam:

GENERAL APPEARANCE AND BEHAVIOR: _____

SPEECH: Normal: ❑ Rate ❑ Rhythm ❑ Latency ❑ Amount ❑ Volume_____

THOUGHT CONTENT: ❑ No SI ❑ No HI ❑ No hallucinations ❑ No delusions

FLOW OF THOUGHT: ❑ Sequential and logical _____

MOOD: _____

AFFECT: _____

INSIGHT: ❑ Poor ❑ Fair ❑ Good _____

JUDGEMENT: ❑ Poor ❑ Fair ❑ Good _____

SENSORIUM/INTELLECT: ❑ A&O × 3 _____

Memory @ 0' _____ 5'_____ Concentration _____ Calculation _____

Assessment & Plan: _____
_____
_____
_____
_____

Dictation job # _____

M.D.: _____ Telephone/Pager # _____

Index